Rx Success™
COMPLETE GUIDE TO MEDICAL MATH

for the

Health Care Professional © 2003

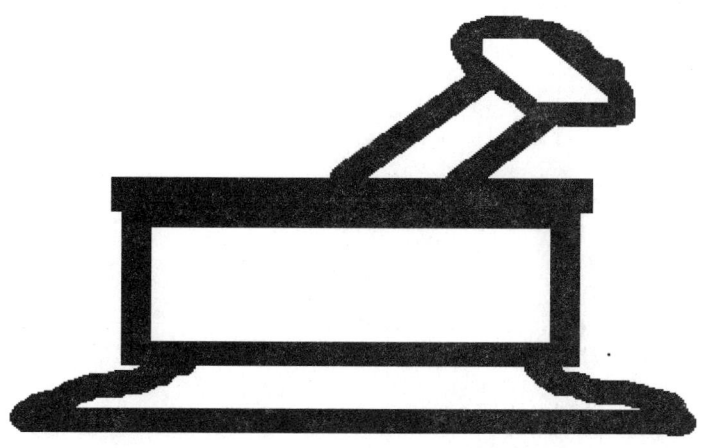

By

Andrea L. Crane

*This book is dedicated to my
wonderful husband, Ken.
Thank you for your understanding,
your support and your ever present help.
I could do nothing without you.*

*Love,
Your Wife*

Rx Success™ Complete Guide to Medical Math

*** *About the Author* ***

Andrea Crane is responsible for the creative vision and technical information which comprise the books, training tools and on-line coursework of the *Rx Success™* Training Program. She brings over twelve years of clinical experience to the *Rx Success™* Program and has worked as a Certified Pharmacy Technician in many different practice settings. Her experience includes positions in hospital, retail, home health care, along with positions in research and educational settings. She attended the University of Colorado at Boulder where she studied Molecular, Cellular and Developmental Biology. She is a state credentialed Pharmacy Technician educator who has taught at a number of community and national vocational education colleges as both full-time and adjunct faculty. She served as the National Curriculum Director for a Pharmacy Technician Training Program and is a current member of the Pharmacy Technician Educators Council. In addition to Exam Preparation tools, Andrea has written several ACPE accredited Continuing Education pieces, and has presented CE for the Colorado Pharmacist's Society Annual Convention. In 1999 Andrea and her husband Kenneth Crane formed **Salt & Light Enterprises, LLC**, a Pharmacy Technician training firm. Andrea currently serves as President of **Salt & Light Enterprises, LLC** and continues to consult for an automation technology company.

Books by Andrea Crane...

- *Rx Success*™ Complete Guide to Medical Math for the Health Care Professional
- *Rx Success*™ National Certification Review Manual for Pharmacy Technicians
- *Rx Success*™ Compounding – Techniques and Theory for the Pharmacy Technician
- *Rx Success*™ Compounding – Techniques and Theory Workbook for the Pharmacy Technician

---

Salt & Light Enterprises, LLC

1004 Mockingbird St.
Brighton, CO 80601

Phone: (866) 898-9374

Web Site: www.rxtechsuccess.com

Email: info@rxtechsuccess.com

All materials contained herein are proprietary and protected under United States Copyright Law.
Rx Success™ *Complete Guide to Medical Math for the Health Care Professional*© Copyright 2003, Salt & Light Enterprises, LLC
Published by: Salt & Light Enterprises, LLC
Brighton, Colorado

Printed in the United States of America

International Standard Book Number: 0-9722464-5-2

Rx Success™ Complete Guide to Medical Math

Foreword...

By far, the most intimidating subject for anyone entering a medical field is math. It is an inescapable reality that medical professionals face on a daily basis. For new students, thoughts of trudging through endless problems are sometimes enough to make an individual reconsider their career options.

This was the reality of medical calculations before Andrea Crane. Math no longer has to be a rigid, unforgiving subject for students. With Andrea's intuitive direction, one can see the approach to a problem with new understanding and clarity. I have had the opportunity to see Andrea in action, teaching students a new approach to problem solving, and have been amazed by the number of people who suddenly find that she has "turned on the light" and the subject is no longer out of their grasp.

Andrea's hands-on approach makes success in this area within everyone's reach. She introduces unique, innovative tools to her students that solidify both concepts and knowledge, but above that, *understanding.* There is a large knowledge gap between having just enough knowledge to pass an exam and having the comprehension to correctly assess daily situations that require calculations.

Andrea has an extraordinary range of pharmacy experience with a diverse and impressive resume of widely varied practice settings. However, she is *driven* by teaching, and has written and developed books, articles and educational tools that have helped thousands of health care professionals achieve success in areas they had failed before. Anyone fortunate enough to find themselves under Andrea's tutelage knows that they are receiving instruction from the absolute best in the industry.

This book was written for every student, regardless of their math background, to produce health care professionals who are both proficient and competent to be an indispensable partner in the health care team.

Heather Caryofilles, PharmD

Rx Success™ Complete Guide to Medical Math

Rx Success™ Complete Guide to Medical Math

Introduction

Dear *Rx Success™* Student:

Welcome to a truly unique way to study Medical Math! I encourage you to take advantage of all of the resources available in this manual. For those of you that cringe at the thought of studying math, this book was written especially for you. We have helped thousands of individuals, just like you, conquer their fear of mathematics and become proficient in Medical Calculations. Every *Rx Success™* learning tool is written with the student in mind and this manual is no exception. Using this manual, you will find that Medical Calculations are easy to learn. Please read the following information to maximize your study time and get everything you can out of this resource.

The Rx Success™ Advantage...

- **Sample Problems** – Each math skill you encounter in this book presents several sample problems. Each sample problem is worked out for you, step by step, complete with explanations of each step. These sample problems serve as guidelines when attempting your own calculations.

- ***Rx Success™ Tutor Sheets™*** – Only *Rx Success™* brings you this exclusive learning tool. There are Tutor Sheets™ available for the most important math skills within this book. Each Tutor Sheet™ guides the student through each step of a calculation, just as if you had your own personal tutor! All of the answers to the Tutor Sheets™ calculations can be found at the bottom of the last sheet. You will use the Sample Problems and the Tutor Sheets™ as examples for performing your own calculations on the homework problems that follow.

- **Homework Problems** – The very best way to master a challenging topic like calculations is clearly to *practice, practice, practice!* The *Rx Success™* manual provides each student with hundreds of homework problems to practice and master these skills. Additionally, the answers to all of these homework problems can be found in the Chapter 16 Answer Key at the back of the book.

Rx Success™ Complete Guide to Medical Math

To achieve success, study each topic in the order presented. First, read about the calculation. Learn to recognize the circumstances under which it is used. Then, follow closely the Sample Problems that are provided. Once you are comfortable with the Sample Problems, move on to the Tutor Sheets™. Fill in the problems, step by step and check your answers at the bottom of these sheets. Finally, you are ready to perform your own calculations by completing the Homework Problems! If you get stuck, refer back to the Sample Problems and Tutor Sheets™ for assistance!

I look forward to your success!

Andrea Crane
Program Director
Rx Success™

Rx Success™ Complete Guide to Medical Math

Table of Contents

Chapter 1 – Getting Started… — Page – 11
- Conversion Factor Quickview — 13
  - Conversion Factor Worksheet — 15
- The "Rules" — 17

Chapter 2 – Roman Numeral Conversions — Page – 21
- Roman Numeral Conversions – Sample Problems — 25
- Roman Numeral Conversions – Homework — 27

Chapter 3 – Military and Standard Time — Page – 31
- Military/Standard Time – Sample Problems — 35
- Military/Standard Time – Homework — 37

Chapter 4 – Temperature Conversions — Page – 41
- Temperature Conversions – Sample Problems — 45
- Temperature Conversions – Tutor Sheets™ — 47
- Temperature Conversions – Homework — 49

Chapter 5 – Metric System Conversions — Page – 51
- Metric System Conversions – Sample Problems — 55
- Metric System Conversions – Tutor Sheets™ — 57
- Metric System Conversions – Homework — 59

Chapter 6 – Fractions/Decimals/Ratios/Percents — Page – 61
- Fractions/Decimals/Ratios/Percents – Sample Problems — 67
- Fractions/Decimals/Ratios/Percents – Tutor Sheets™ — 69
- Fractions/Decimals/Ratios/Percents – Homework — 71

Chapter 7 – Cross Multiplication — Page – 73
- Cross Multiplication – Sample Problems — 79
- Cross Multiplication – Tutor Sheets™ — 83
- Cross Multiplication – Homework — 87

Chapter 8 – Apothecary, Metric, Household Conversions — Page – 91
- Apothecary, Metric, Household Conversions – Sample Problems — 95
- Apothecary, Metric, Household Conversions – Tutor Sheets™ — 99
- Apothecary, Metric, Household Conversions – Homework — 103

Rx Success™ Complete Guide to Medical Math

Chapter 9 – Dosage Calculations — Page – 109
- Step One – Calculating Volume — 111
  - Dosage Calculations – Sample Problems — 113
  - Dosage Calculations – Tutor Sheets™ — 115
  - Dosage Calculations – Homework — 119

- Step Two – Calculating Doses Using Body Weight — 125
  - Dosage Calculations – Sample Problems — 127
  - Dosage Calculations – Tutor Sheets™ — 131
  - Dosage Calculations – Homework — 139

Chapter 10 – Insulin Calculations — Page – 149
- Insulin Calculations – Sample Problems — 155
- Insulin Calculations – Tutor Sheets™ — 157
- Insulin Calculations – Homework — 163

Chapter 11 – Percent Solutions — Page – 169
- Percent Solutions – Sample Problems — 175
- Percent Solutions – Tutor Sheets™ — 179
- Percent Solutions – Homework — 183

Chapter 12 – IV Drip Rate Calculations — Page – 187
- IV Solutions — 189
- IV Drip Rate Calculations — 193
  - IV Drip Rate Calculations – Sample Problems — 197
  - IV Drip Rate Calculations – Tutor Sheets™ — 205
  - IV Drip Rate Calculations – Homework — 211

Chapter 13 – Alligations — Page – 227
- Alligations – Sample Problems — 231
- Alligations – Tutor Sheets™ — 237
- Alligations – Homework — 241

Chapter 14 – Pediatric Dosage Calculations — Page – 247
- Pediatric Dosage Calculations – Sample Problems — 253
- Pediatric Dosage Calculations – Tutor Sheets™ — 255
- Pediatric Dosage Calculations – Homework — 257

Chapter 15 – Pharmaco-Economic Calculations — Page – 265
- Pharmaco-Economics – Sample Problems — 271
- Pharmaco-Economics – Tutor Sheets™ — 279
- Pharmaco-Economics – Homework — 283

Chapter 16 – Homework Answer Key — Page – 295

Rx Success™ Complete Guide to Medical Math

Chapter One

Getting Started...

Rx Success™ Complete Guide to Medical Math

Conversion Factor Quickview

The following conversion equivalents integrate Household, Metric and Apothecary measurement systems. As a result of this integration, these conversions are approximate but accepted equivalents

Pharmacy Conversion Factors		
1 dr	4 ml (cc)	
1 pt	16 oz	480 ml (cc)
1 qt	1 L	2 pt
1 lb	16 oz	454 g
1 gal	4 qt, 4 L	4000 ml (cc)
1 gr	60 mg	
1 g	15 gr	1000 mg
1 oz	8 dr	30 ml (cc)
1 tsp (t)	5 ml (cc)	
1 T	3 tsp	15 ml (cc)
1 kg	2.2 lb	

Abbreviations	
dr	dram
g	gram
gal	gallon
gr	grain
kg	kilogram
L	liter
lb	pound
ml	milliliter
oz	ounce
pt	pint
qt	quart
T, tbsp	tablespoon
t, tsp	teaspoon

Temperature Conversions

Celsius = 0.56 (Fahrenheit − 32)

Fahrenheit = (Celsius X 1.8) + 32

Rx Success™ Complete Guide to Medical Math

Conversion Factor Worksheet

Fill in the correct conversion "codes" for the following equivalents. These are all equivalents that should be memorized.

1) 1 kg = _____ lb

2) 1 oz = _____ ml

3) 1 T = _____ ml

4) 1 gr = _____ mg

5) 1 L = _____ qt

6) 1 pt = _____ ml

7) 1 t = _____ ml

8) 1 pt = _____ oz

9) 1 qt = _____ pt

10) 1 lb = _____ g

Rx Success™ Complete Guide to Medical Math

Rx Success™ Complete Guide to Medical Math

The "Rules"

Please read the following information very carefully. When performing medical calculations, accuracy is always a primary concern. However, inherent inconsistencies do exist. You will find explanations for some of the most common inconsistencies, below, as well as the correct way to deal with these problems.

Rounding:
Students of math always want to know the rules on rounding. "Do I round up or leave it? When do I round? How many numbers do I leave?" These simple rules will provide guidance when dealing with these very important questions.

- ✓ Round up or leave as is? First, identify how many decimal places you want in the number. For example, we will use two decimal places. Before we round, the number looks like this:

    31.02874

    Since we only want two decimal places, the "2" is the number that we will either leave as is or round up. Whether to round up or not is dependant on the number to the immediate right of the "2". If this number is a "5" or higher, we will round up and replace the "2" with a "3". Since the number *is* greater than "5", we will round up. The correctly rounded number now looks like this:

    31.03

    If the number to the immediate right of the "2" had been a "4" or lower, (for example: 31.02193) we would have left the "2" and the correctly rounded number would have looked like this:

    31.02

- ✓ When do I round? This rule is simple. Try not to round until the very last step of the problem, when the final answer is obtained. If a problem takes three or four steps to complete and the answers are rounded after each step, this will diminish the accuracy of the final answer. Each time an answer is rounded, accuracy is lost because numbers are dropped from the exact answer. Therefore, it is good practice to try not to round any numbers except the final answer.

- ✓ How many numbers do I leave? To answer this question, the purpose of those numbers must be understood. Remember that each decimal place represents increased accuracy. For example, assume that the final answer to a dosage calculation problem is

    4.2783951 ml

    Think about this, if you were asked to pour out 4.2783951 mls from a bottle of liquid, could you do it? Of course not! There are simply too many decimal places. We cannot accurately measure to that many decimal places! However, if we were to round this number to two decimal places (**4.28 mls**), we could accurately measure this amount. This means that the accuracy of the number is only as good as our ability to measure the quantity accurately! *As a general rule,* ***two decimal places*** *are usually as close as we can accurately measure with the graduated devices found in a medical setting.*

The 10% Rule:
The "10% Rule" says that when calculating dosage strengths, as long as we are accurate to within 10% (10% error or less), the therapeutics of the drug on the body will remain the same. This is not to be used as a "catch all" excuse to make mistakes! Rather, the 10% Rule covers two people who are performing the same calculation by different methods. The two individuals will not likely come up with *precisely* the same answer. However, as long as each party performed the calculation correctly, their answers should be within 10% of each other and therefore, therapeutically equivalent. Read the section below (Discrepancies in Medical Conversions) for a general understanding of why these discrepancies occur.

Discrepancies in Medical Conversions:
As you become more familiar with medical math, you will probably begin to realize that there are "discrepancies" between references about some conversion factors (codes) or that you get slightly different answers than someone else or this book. For instance, take the conversion factor for "mg" and "grains". Some references say that 60 mg = 1 grain. For every book that says 60 mg, you will find another that says 65 mg = 1 grain. As you continue through the math, you will find many more of these "discrepancies". Medicine is littered with them! Another instance is with pint bottles of fluids. Some pint bottles say "**473 mL**", and some say "**480 mL**". And to confuse matters even further, it is a commonly used conversion that 1L = 1qt. This means that if 2 pt = 1 qt then 2 pt *also equals* 1 L. We also know that 1000 ml = 1 L, so we can correctly assume that 2 pt = 1000 ml. So there must be **500 mL in 1 pt**. So, we have this "discrepancy" that encompasses values anywhere from 473 mL to 500 mL and they ALL are supposed to equal one pint! This brings us to the question of accurately performing medical calculations because we all know that patient safety depends upon accuracy! Suppose one person is using 473 ml = 1 pt and another is using 480 mL = 1 pt, they obviously will not get the same answer. But in medicine we are given a "10% Rule". This says that as long as we are accurate to within 10% (10% error or less), the therapeutics of the drug on the body will not change. Looking at the conversion factors for mg and grain (60 mg vs. 65 mg), the 5 mg difference will give a discrepancy of up to 8%, so either 60 mg OR 65 mg is an acceptable equivalent for one grain.

The other reason for these discrepancies is that there are many different number systems that are used in medical math. Here is a partial list of some of the most commonly used.

1. **Avoir-Dupois and Troy Systems** – The avoir-dupois is a French system of measurement, literally meaning "goods having weight". There are "avoir-dupois pounds" and "avoir-dupois ounces", etc. This system

is based on the following equivalents: 28 grams = 1 oz (avoir-dupois) and 16 oz (avoir-dupois) = 1 lb (avoir-dupois) and represents the pounds and ounces that we are familiar with in the United States. These are the same pounds and ounces used in the English system. Additionally, these same units are used in the Troy system of measurement. There are Troy ounces and Troy pounds. For example, 1 avoir-dupois ounce = 0.911 Troy ounces. Here are some equivalents from both the avoir-dupois and the Troy systems of measurement.

Avoirdupois System
- 1 pound = 16 ounces
- 1 ounce = 16 dram
- 1 drachma = 4 quarters

In the Troy System:
- 1 pound = 12 ounces
- 1 Troy ounce = 8 Troy drams
- 1 dram = 3 scruples
- 1 scruple = 20 grains

2. **Apothecary System** – This system, like other, older systems of measurement is slowly being phased out. Yet in medicine we still use Apothecary units like grains, minims and drams. Roman numerals, rather than Arabic numbers, are commonly seen in the Apothecary system.

3. **Metric System** – The Metric system uses base units of grams, liters and meters to represent dry weight, volume (liquid measurements) and length, respectively. The Metric system uses prefixes (i.e. milli-, micro-, kilo-, centi-) to denote multipliers of "10" on each unit. The same prefixes are used for each of the three base units.

4. **Household** – The household system of measurement uses mainly avoir-dupois units like pounds and ounces and also quarts, gallons and pints. Household measurements also include common medication administration units such as teaspoons and tablespoons.

5. **English** – This system is still firmly entrenched in the United States. Using such length measurements as miles, furlongs, fathoms, yards and inches.

You can see from this small sampling of measurement systems how terribly confusing it would be to have to memorize every conversion between all the systems in the world. That is why, around the world, the Metric System is the primary system of measurement that is used. However, in medicine, there are still units from these other systems that are commonly used. Because of the integration between these measurement systems, numbers must be rounded here and there to produce numbers that practitioners are able to work with and remember. Rounding in this way can cause discrepancies among two people calculating for the very same value!

Decimals

"Implied Decimals" – Even though whole numbers are not written with decimal points, they all have one! Even though it is not convention to write in a decimal point on a whole number like 1,170 it is there. In this case the decimal is to the immediate right of the "0".

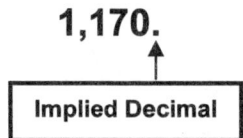

You must know how to recognize the placement of the decimal in whole numbers when doing metric conversions and various other types of problems.

"Naked Decimals" – A naked decimal occurs when a number is written with a decimal as the first character written on the furthest left side of the number. For example

.25

This decimal is considered "naked" because it is not flanked by a number on the left side. For the sake of clarity, in medicine all decimals *must* be flanked on either side by a number. The number that must be placed on the left side of a naked decimal is "zero". A zero in this position will not change the value of the number, rather, it simply emphasizes the fact that a decimal is there. The importance of this practice can be seen in the following physician's order.

Order: .25 mg of drug

Suppose the physician was writing quickly and neglected to make sure that the decimal point was clear enough to be read. The order now looks like this.

Order: 25 mg of drug

The patient would receive a 100 fold overdose of this medication! Therefore all naked decimals must be covered with a zero on the left side. This way, even if the decimal point were not clearly visible, the zero would draw attention to the fact that a decimal is, indeed, present.

Order: 0.25 mg of drug

Rx Success™ Complete Guide to Medical Math

Chapter Two

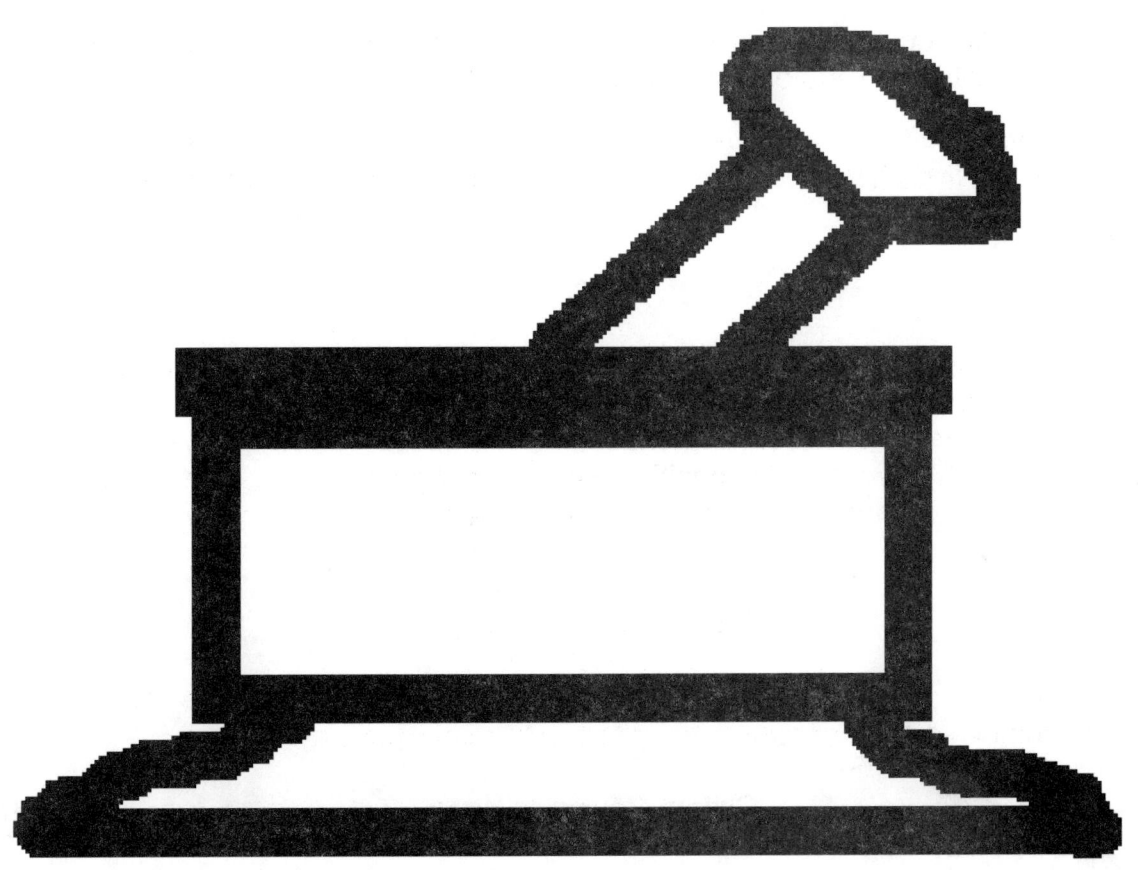

Roman Numeral Conversions

Roman Numeral Conversions

The ancient Romans did not have unique symbols that represented numbers. Instead, they used letters to represent numerical values. They assigned numerical values to certain letters (i.e. I, V, X, L, C, D, M). This allowed them to put together combinations of letters to represent all the numbers not given a single letter designation.

The major differences between Roman and Arabic numerals (which are used today) are that the ancient Romans did not have a symbol for zero, and that the placement of the letters within the entire number can either indicate subtraction or addition.

Here is a list of the seven letters that are used with their respective, assigned values.

Roman Numeral	Arabic Number
I	1
V	5
X	10
L	50
C	100
D	500
M	1000

There are several rules governing the placement of letters. Read these carefully and use them to complete the homework that follows. Although you will rarely use Roman Numerals, you will occasionally see them show up on prescriptions. They are sometimes used to express dates and when denoting the DEA schedule given to medications.

1. When a letter is repeated, its value is repeated.
   - II = 2
   - VII = 7
   - XX = 20

2. When a letter of smaller value is placed after a letter of larger value, the smaller is added to the larger numeral.
   - VI = 6
   - XI = 11
   - XV = 15
   - CL = 150
   - MC = 1100

Rx Success™ Complete Guide to Medical Math

3. When a letter of smaller value is placed before a letter of larger value, the smaller value is subtracted from the larger value.
   - IV = 4
   - IX = 9
   - XC = 90

4. A letter cannot be repeated more than three times.
   - IIII is NOT 4
   - IV = 4
   - XXXX is NOT 40
   - XL = 40

5. V, L and D are never repeated.
   - VV is NOT 10
   - X = 10
   - LL is NOT 100
   - C = 100
   - DD is NOT 1000
   - M = 1000

6. V, L and D are never subtracted from larger numerals.
   - VX is NOT 5
   - V = 5
   - LC is NOT 50
   - L = 50
   - DM is NOT 500
   - D = 500

7. Never subtract more than one numeral.
   - IIV is NOT 3
   - III = 3
   - XXL is NOT 30
   - XXX = 30

8. Use I only before V and X (only the next two higher value numerals). Use X only before L and C. Use C only before D and M.
   - IV = 4
   - IX = 9
   - IC is NOT 99
   - XLV = 45
   - XC = 90
   - XM is NOT 990

Page - 24

Rx Success™ Complete Guide to Medical Math

Roman Numeral Conversions – Sample Problems

Here is a list of Roman Numerals and their Arabic equivalents:

Arabic Number	Roman Numeral
1	I
2	II
3	III
4	IV
5	V
6	VI
7	VII
8	VIII
9	IX
10	X
20	XX
50	L
100	C
500	D
1000	M

Note: Use these values to do the homework on the next page.

Roman Numeral Conversions - Homework

Write the Roman Numeral equivalents for the following numbers:

Arabic Number	Roman Numeral
1. 4	IV
2. 10	X
3. 18	
4. 23	
5. 9	
6. 14	
7. 11	
8. 27	
9. 19	
10. 30	
11. 54	
12. 25	
13. 16	
14. 45	
15. 50	
16. 32	
17. 101	
18. 109	
19. 75	

Rx Success™ Complete Guide to Medical Math

Arabic Number	Roman Numeral
20. 84	
21. 93	
22. 275	
23. 153	
24. 400	
25. 323	
26. 450	
27. 501	
28. 87	
29. 615	
30. 231	
31. 870	
32. 500	
33. 790	
34. 425	
35. 1250	
36. 764	
37. 123	
38. 1500	
39. 2000	
40. 2003	

Rx Success™ Complete Guide to Medical Math

Write the Arabic Number equivalents for the following Roman Numerals:

Arabic Number	Roman Numeral
1.	VII
2.	III
3.	IX
4.	XI
5.	CX
6.	MCM
7.	XL
8.	LX
9.	CD
10.	DCXVII
11.	LXXXIV
12.	MMIII
13.	MCMLXXII
14.	LVII
15.	CXXIII
16.	XIX
17.	DC
18.	XCIV
19.	CLXXXVI
20.	CMXCIX

Rx Success™ Complete Guide to Medical Math

Chapter Three

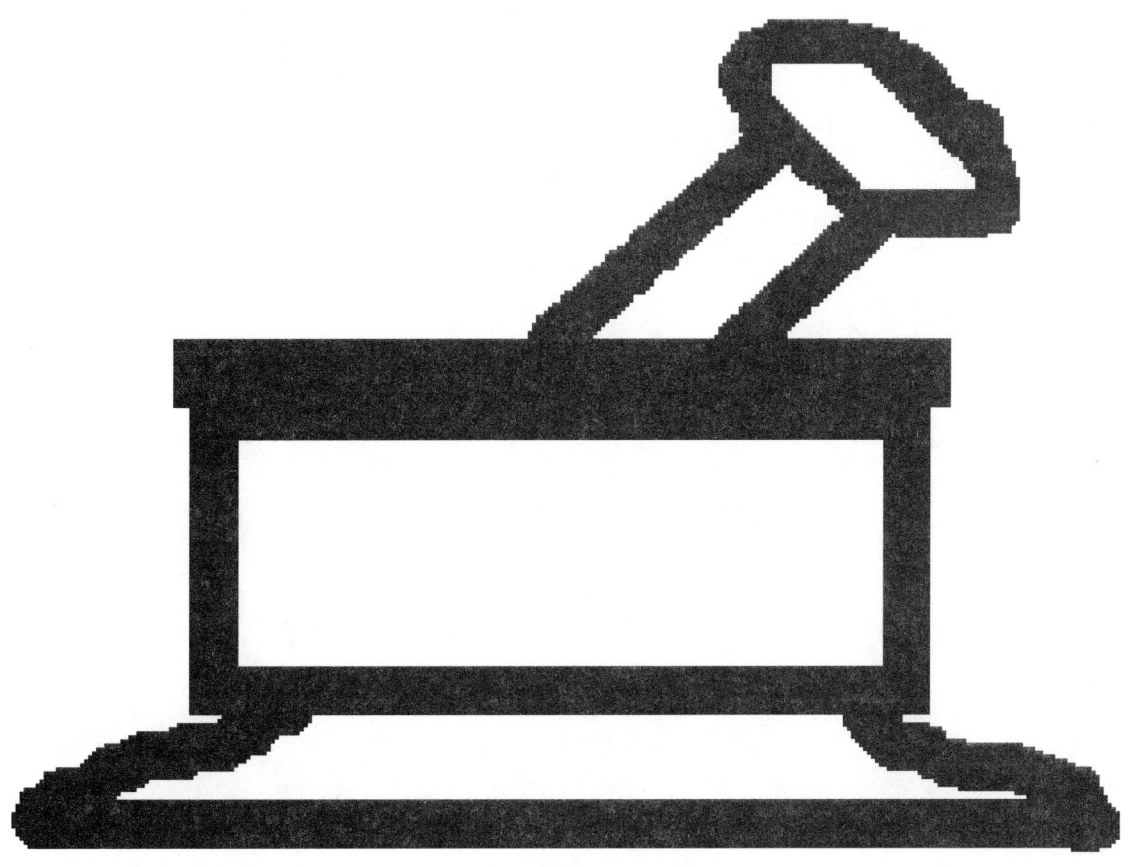

Military and Standard Time

Rx Success™ Complete Guide to Medical Math

Military and Standard Time

Military time (24-hour time) is exclusively used in hospitals. Suppose a hospital physician writes an order for a medication to be given at 4:00. Since hospitals care for acutely ill people, medications are given around the clock. So, is this medication to be given at 4:00 AM or 4:00 PM? The use of military time solves this problem.

Military time uses a 24 hour clock rather than the standard 12 hour clock. On a standard clock, 4:00 AM looks exactly like 4:00 PM. The advantage of using military time is that no two times during a 24 hour day are the same. Assuming the day begins at 12:01 AM, (in military time, this is 0001 hours) and the day ends at 12:00 midnight (in military time, this is 2400 hours), there are a total of 24 hours in between. Look at the table below to see how military time corresponds to standard time during that 24 hour period.

Standard	*Military*
1:00 AM	0100 hours
2:00 AM	0200 hours
3:00 AM	0300 hours
4:00 AM	0400 hours
5:00 AM	0500 hours
6:00 AM	0600 hours
7:00 AM	0700 hours
8:00 AM	0800 hours
9:00 AM	0900 hours
10:00 AM	1000 hours
11:00 AM	1100 hours
12:00 Noon	1200 hours
1:00 PM	1300 hours
2:00 PM	1400 hours
3:00 PM	1500 hours
4:00 PM	1600 hours
5:00 PM	1700 hours
6:00 PM	1800 hours
7:00 PM	1900 hours
8:00 PM	2000 hours
9:00 PM	2100 hours
10:00 PM	2200 hours
11:00 PM	2300 hours
12:00 Midnight	2400 hours

Rx Success™ Complete Guide to Medical Math

Military/Standard Time – Sample Problems

Study the following sample problems. Then, continue on to the Military/Standard Time Homework.

1. Convert 3:30 pm into Military Time.

Since 3:30 pm is *after* noon, we must add 12 hours to the time.

3:30 + 12 hours = 15:30 hours

Now, drop the colon in the middle and the answer is **1530 hours (fifteen *hundred* and thirty hours).**

---

2. Convert 7:22 am into Military Time.

Since 7:22 am is *before* noon, we simply remove the colon, and the answer is **0722 hours (oh seven *hundred* and twenty-two hours).**

---

3. Convert 10:15 pm into Military Time

Since 10:15 pm is *after* noon, we must add 12 hours to the time.

10:15 + 12 hours = 22:15 hours

Now, drop the colon in the middle and the answer is **2215 hours (twenty-two *hundred* and fifteen hours).**

Rx Success™ Complete Guide to Medical Math

Military/Standard Time - Homework

By using military time in a hospital setting, there is never any confusion as to whether a drug is to be given in the AM or PM. Try the following problems to make sure you can convert back and forth.

Convert the following Standard Times to Military:

Standard	Military
1. 1:00 AM	
2. 2:00 AM	
3. 3:00 AM	
4. 4:00 AM	
5. 5:00 AM	
6. 6:00 AM	
7. 7:00 AM	
8. 8:00 AM	
9. 9:00 AM	
10. 10:00 AM	
11. 11:00 AM	
12. 12:00 Noon	
13. 1:00 PM	
14. 2:00 PM	
15. 3:00 PM	
16. 4:00 PM	
17. 5:00 PM	
18. 6:00 PM	
19. 7:00 PM	
20. 8:00 PM	
21. 9:00 PM	
22. 10:00 PM	
23. 11:00 PM	
24. 12:00 Midnight	
25. 1:31 AM	
26. 12:17 PM	
27. 8:30 PM	

Rx Success™ Complete Guide to Medical Math

Standard	Military
28. 3:23 PM	
29. 9:18 AM	
30. 1:10 PM	
31. 8:30 AM	
32. 7:55 PM	
33. 3:15 AM	
34. 7:45 AM	
35. 10:32 PM	
36. 11:57 AM	
37. 11:20 PM	
38. 6:30 PM	
39. 5:45 PM	
40. 2:30 PM	

Convert the following Military Times to Standard:

Military	Standard
1. 1200 hours	
2. 1300 hours	
3. 1400 hours	
4. 1500 hours	
5. 1600 hours	
6. 1700 hours	
7. 1800 hours	
8. 1900 hours	
9. 2000 hours	
10. 2100 hours	
11. 2200 hours	
12. 2300 hours	
13. 2400 hours	
14. 0100 hours	
15. 0200 hours	

Rx Success™ Complete Guide to Medical Math

Military	Standard
16. 0300 hours	
17. 0400 hours	
18. 0500 hours	
19. 0600 hours	
20. 0700 hours	
21. 0800 hours	
22. 0900 hours	
23. 1000 hours	
24. 1100 hours	
25. 0001 hours	
26. 1625 hours	
27. 0315 hours	
28. 2245 hours	
29. 2030 hours	
30. 1156 hours	
31. 1201 hours	
32. 1925 hours	
33. 0745 hours	
34. 0902 hours	
35. 1250 hours	
36. 2145 hours	
37. 2318 hours	
38. 0620 hours	
39. 1745 hours	
40. 1430 hours	

Rx Success™ Complete Guide to Medical Math

Chapter Four

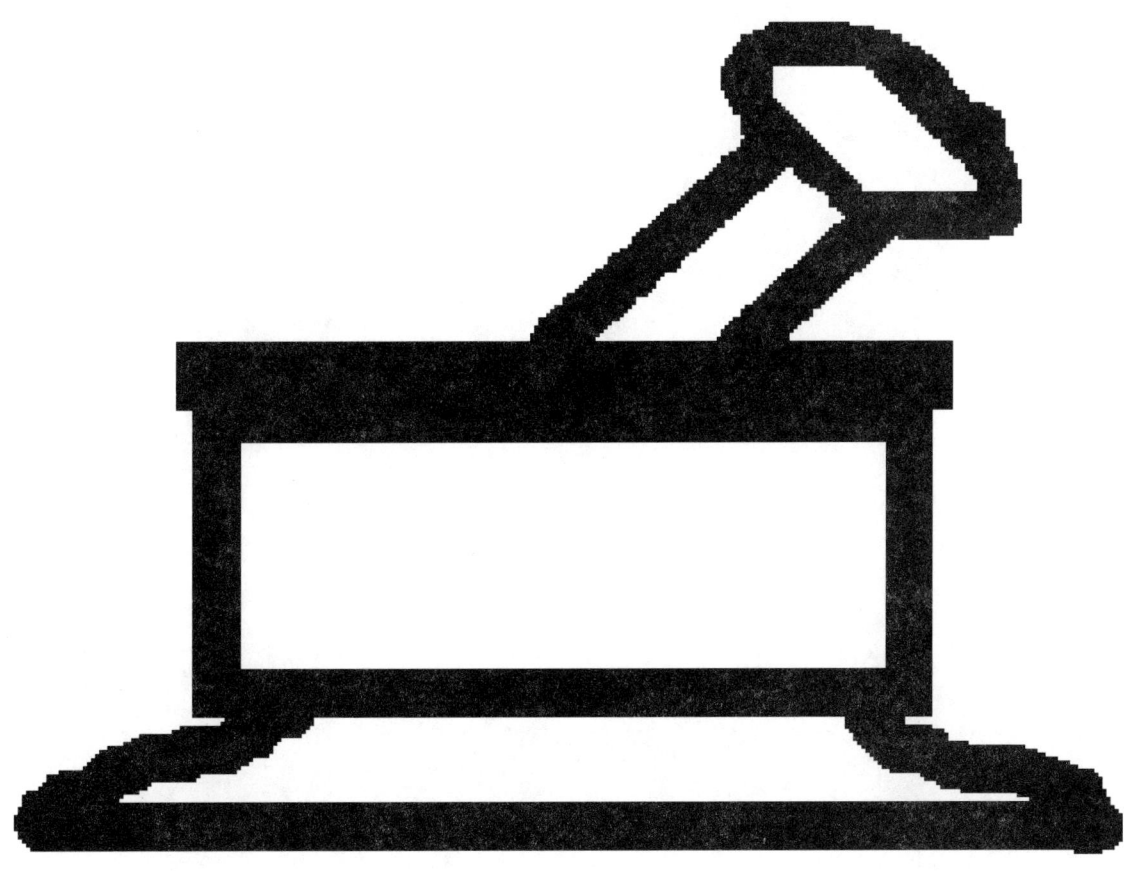

Temperature Conversions

Rx Success™ Complete Guide to Medical Math

Temperature Conversions

Most temperatures, in this country, are measured in Fahrenheit degrees (F°). However, much of the literature containing specific drug storage requirements measures temperature in Celsius degrees (C°). To ensure proper storage for medications, health care professionals must be able to convert back and forth between Fahrenheit and Celsius. There are two formulas to use for these conversions. The one used depends on whether the need is to convert to Fahrenheit or Celsius.

- **C° = 0.55 (F° - 32)**
  Use this formula to convert **from F° to C°**.

- **F° = (C° x 1.8) + 32**
  Use this formula to convert **from C° to F°**.

Study closely the sample problems that follow and then complete the Temperature Conversion Tutor Sheets™. This will provide a good background for the Homework problems at the end of this chapter!

Rx Success™ Complete Guide to Medical Math

Temperature Conversions – Sample Problems

1. **Convert 80° F to C°.** First, determine which of the previous formulas to use. Since we are converting **from** F° **to** C°, we will use the first formula. Simply plug the F° value (which is 80) into the equation. It will look like this:

    C° = 0.55 (80 - 32)

    First, do the operation in the parentheses (80 – 32 = 48). Then, multiply the answer by 0.55 (48 x 0.55 = **26.4° C**).

2. **Convert 23° F to C°.** We will use the same formula to solve this one. Plug in the F° value as before. The equation will look like this:

    C° = 0.55 (23 - 32)

    First, do the operation in the parentheses (23 – 32 = -9). Then, multiply the answer by 0.55 (-9 x 0.55 = **-5° C**).

3. **Convert 14° C to F°.** Since we are converting **from** C° **to** F°, we will use the second formula. This time, plug the C° value into the equation. It will look like this:

    F° = (14 x 1.8) + 32

    First, do the operation in the parentheses (14 x 1.8 = 25.2). Then, add 32 to the answer (25.2 + 32 = **57.2° F**).

4. **Convert –36° C to F°.** We will again use the second formula to calculate this temperature conversion. The formula looks like this:

    F° = (-36 x 1.8) + 32

    First, do the operation in the parentheses (-36 x 1.8 = -64.8). Then, add 32 to the answer (-64.8 + 32 = **-32.8° F**).

It is also useful to know the proper temperature ranges for different medication storage requirements. Familiarize yourself with the table that follows for this information.

Storage Temperature Requirements

Storage Type	Celsius Range	Fahrenheit Range
Incubator or Warmer	30° and 40° C	86° and 104° F
Room Temperature	15° and 30° C	59° and 86° F
Refrigerated	2° and 8° C	36° and 46° F
Freezer	-20° and -10° C	-4° and 14° F

Rx Success™ Complete Guide to Medical Math

Temperature Conversions - *Tutor Sheets*™

USE THIS WORKSHEET AS A GUIDE TO HELP YOU SOLVE THE HOMEWORK PROBLEMS!

1. 68° F = _____ ° C

    a) C° = 0.55 (____ - 32)

    b) ____ - 32 = ____

    c) ____ x 0.55 = ____

    Formula
    C° = 0.55 (F° - 32)

2. -12° F = _____ ° C

    a) C° = 0.55 (____ - 32)

    b) ____ - 32 = ____

    c) ____ x 0.55 = ____

    Formula
    C° = 0.55 (F° - 32)

3. 70° C = _____ ° F

    a) F° = (____ x 1.8) + 32

    b) ____ x 1.8 = ____

    c) ____ + 32 = ____

    Formula
    F° = (C° x 1.8) + 32

4. 25° C = _____ ° F

    a) F° = (____ x 1.8) + 32

    b) ____ x 1.8 = ____

    c) ____ + 32 = ____

    Formula
    F° = (C° x 1.8) + 32

Rx Success™ Complete Guide to Medical Math

5. 106° C = _____ ° F   **Formula**

   a)

   b)

   c)

6. 30° F = _____ ° C   **Formula**

   a)

   b)

   c)

7. 112° F = _____ ° C   **Formula**

   a)

   b)

   c)

8. -20° C = _____ ° F   **Formula**

   a)

   b)

   c)

Answers to Tutor Sheets™ Calculations
1) 19.8° C   2) -24.2° C   3) 158° F   4) 77° F   5) 222.8° F   6) -1.1° C   7) 44° C   8) -4° F

Rx Success™ Complete Guide to Medical Math

Temperature Conversions - Homework

Convert the following temperatures to C° or F°:

Celsius	Fahrenheit
1. 31° C	
2.	120° F
3.	16° F
4. 100° C	
5.	72° F
6. 89° C	
7. 17° C	
8.	100° F
9.	32° F
10.	0° F
11. 23.5° C	
12.	-12° F
13. -15° C	
14. 98.5° C	
15.	97° F
16.	98.6° F
17. 2° C	
18.	14° F
19. 8° C	
20. 40° C	
21. 30° C	
22.	60° F
23.	212° F
24.	86° F

Rx Success™ Complete Guide to Medical Math

Celsius	Fahrenheit
25. 15° C	
26. -50° C	
27.	104° F
28. 0° C	
29.	-4° F
30. -20° C	

Rx Success™ Complete Guide to Medical Math

Chapter Five

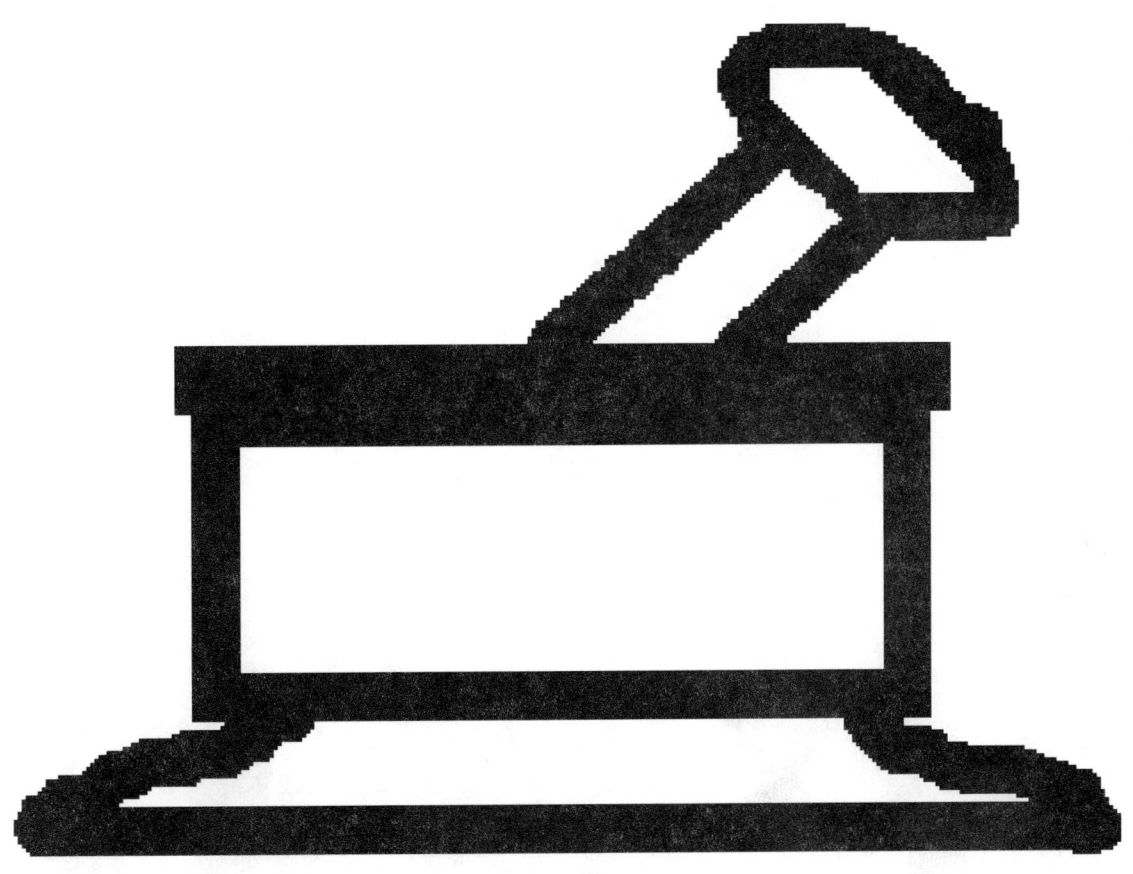

Metric System Conversions

Rx Success™ Complete Guide to Medical Math

Metric System Conversions

All health care professionals must be able to convert back and forth among metric units within the same "family". Prefixes are added to make the base units of these families smaller or larger. The largest unit that we will work with gets a prefix of, kilo-. The smallest unit we will work with gets a prefix of, micro-. Here are the prefixes in order of largest to smallest.

kilo- _____ _____ base unit _____ _____ milli- _____ _____ micro-

The blank spaces between the units have prefixes as well, however, they are not important for our study.

The metric system has three "families" of measurement.

1. **Metric Unit of Length** – The base unit of length in the metric system is the **meter**. For frame of reference, a meter is about the same length as a yard. When the prefixes are added, the metric family of length measurement looks like this: (the abbreviations are directly under the units)

kilometer ____ ____ meter ____ ____ millimeter ____ ____ micrometer
(km) (m) (mm) (mcm)

2. **Metric Unit of Dry Weight** – The base unit of dry weight in the metric system is the **gram**. The weight of a gram is roughly equal to ten small paperclips. When the prefixes are added, the metric family of dry weight measurement looks like this: (the abbreviations are directly under the units)

kilogram ____ ____ gram ____ ____ milligram ____ ____ microgram
(kg) (g) (mg) (mcg)

3. **Metric Unit of Liquid Volume** – The base unit of liquid volume in the metric system is the **liter**. The volume of a liter is exactly one-half of a two-liter of soda, or about a quarter of a gallon. When the prefixes are added, the metric family of liquid volume measurement looks like this: (the abbreviations are directly under the units)

kiloliter ____ ____ liter ____ ____ milliliter ____ ____ microliter
(kL) (L) (mL) (mcL)

Rx Success™ Complete Guide to Medical Math

Assume there are **three** spaces in between the prefixes. To convert back and forth within a family, just move the decimal the required number of spaces. You will always move the decimal in multiples of three spaces (three, six or nine spaces).

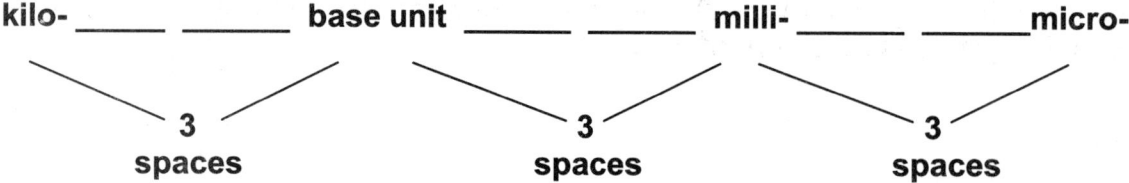

To move from **kilo-** to the **base unit** requires a move of three spaces. **Micro-** to the **base unit** requires a move of six spaces. To move from **kilo-** to **micro-** requires a move of nine spaces, and so on.

To determine which direction to move the decimal (right or left), simply look at the chart. For instance, if converting kg to g, see that if we begin at **kilo-**, to get to **gram (or, the base unit)** you must move three spaces to the right. Remember, if the number does not already contain a decimal, it is <u>always</u> to the right of the last digit. Look over the following Sample Problems and Tutor Sheets™ and then begin the Metric Conversion Homework at the end of this section. Use the conversion charts to help you figure how many places to move the decimal and in which direction.

*Note: Never leave a decimal "naked" on the left side of a number. *Always* place a zero to the left of the decimal!*

Incorrect: .38   **Correct: 0.38**

Rx Success™ Complete Guide to Medical Math

Metric System Conversions - Sample Problems

1. 30 kg = _____ g

To convert from kg to g, move the decimal three places to the right. The decimal originates to the right of the zero.

30.⌣⌣⌣

Fill in the spaces with zeros...

30 0 0 0.   So...

30 kg = **30,000 g**

---

2. 30 kg = _____ mg

To convert from kg to mg, move the decimal six places to the right. The decimal originates to the right of the zero.

30.⌣⌣⌣⌣⌣⌣

Fill in the spaces with zeros...

30 0 0 0 0 0 0.

30 kg = **30,000,000 mg**

---

3. 4.5 L = _____ ml

To convert from L to mL, move the decimal three places to the right.

4.5⌣⌣⌣.

Fill in the spaces with zeros...

4.5 0 0 0.

4.5 L = **4,500 ml**

Rx Success™ Complete Guide to Medical Math

4. 370 cc = _____ L

Keep in mind, a "cc" is the same thing as a "ml". To convert from ml to L, move the decimal three places to the left.

.370.   So…

370 ml = **.370 L**

However, our decimal is "naked" and we have an unecessary zero in the furthest right position. To correct…

370 ml = **0.37 L**

---

5. 2700 mg = _____ g

To convert from mg to g, move the decimal three places to the left.

2.700.

2700 mg = **2.700 g**

Remove the two unnecessary zeros from the right side of the answer.

2700 mg = **2.7 g**

Rx Success™ Complete Guide to Medical Math

Metric System Conversions - *Tutor Sheets*™

USE THIS WORKSHEET AS A GUIDE TO HELP YOU SOLVE THE HOMEWORK PROBLEMS!

Formula
kilo- ____ ____ base unit ____ ____ milli- ____ ____ micro-

1. 890.3 g = __890,300__ mg
   a) Going from **gram** to **mg**
   b) Move decimal **three** places to the **right**
   c) 890.3 g = __ __ __ , __ __ __ mg

2. 23,895 mcl = __0.023895__ L
   a) Going from _____ to _____
   b) Move decimal _____ places to the _____
   c) 23,895 mcl = __ . __ __ __ __ __ __ L

3. 0.00785 kg = __7850__ mg
   a) Going from _____ to _____
   b) Move decimal _____ places to the _____
   c) 0.00785 kg = __ , __ __ __ mg

4. 8,590 cc = __8.59__ L
   a) Going from _____ to _____
   b) Move decimal _____ places to the _____
   c) 8,590 ml = __ . __ __ __ L

5. 0.275 kg = __275__ g
   a) Going from _____ to _____

Page - 57

b) Move decimal _____ places to the _____
c) 0.275 kg = __ __ __ g

Answers to Tutor Sheets™ Calculations
1) 890,300 mg   2) 0.023895 L   3) 7850 mg   4) 8.59 L   5) 275 g

Rx Success™ Complete Guide to Medical Math
Metric Conversions - Homework

Metric Measure of Dry Weight: Fill in the metric equivalents for the given weight values. Use number one as an example.

	mcg	mg	g	kg
1.	815,500	**815.5**	0.8155	0.0008155
2.		**750**		
3.	**82.3**			
4.			**0.0045**	
5.				**1.12**
6.		**0.75**		
7.			**45**	
8.				**0.00025**
9.		**125**		
10.		**0.075**		
11.			**105**	
12.				**1.0075**
13.				**10.2**
14.		**10,000**		
15.			**950**	

Metric Measure of Volume: Fill in the metric equivalents for the given liquid, volume values. Use number one as an example.

	mcl	ml	L	kl
1.	62,500	**62.5**	0.0625	0.0000625
2.		**70**		
3.		**190**		
4.			**1.2**	
5.		**31.05**		
6.		**0.075**		
7.				**0.00875**
8.				**0.00015**

Rx Success™ Complete Guide to Medical Math

mcl	ml	L	kl
9.		7.024	
10.		0.00205	
11.		10	
12.			0.208
13.			1
14.	8.0005		
15.		2.03	

Metric Measure of Length: Fill in the metric equivalents for the given length values. Use number one as an example.

mcm	mm	m	km
1. 700,000	700	0.7	0.0007
2.			0.0000085
3. 115,000			
4.		0.00125	
5.			1.12
6.	0.815		
7.		9.1	
8.			0.00025
9.			6.05
10. 900			
11.		7	
12.			0.010205
13.			0.004
14.	127,500		
15.	425		

Rx Success™ Complete Guide to Medical Math

Chapter Six

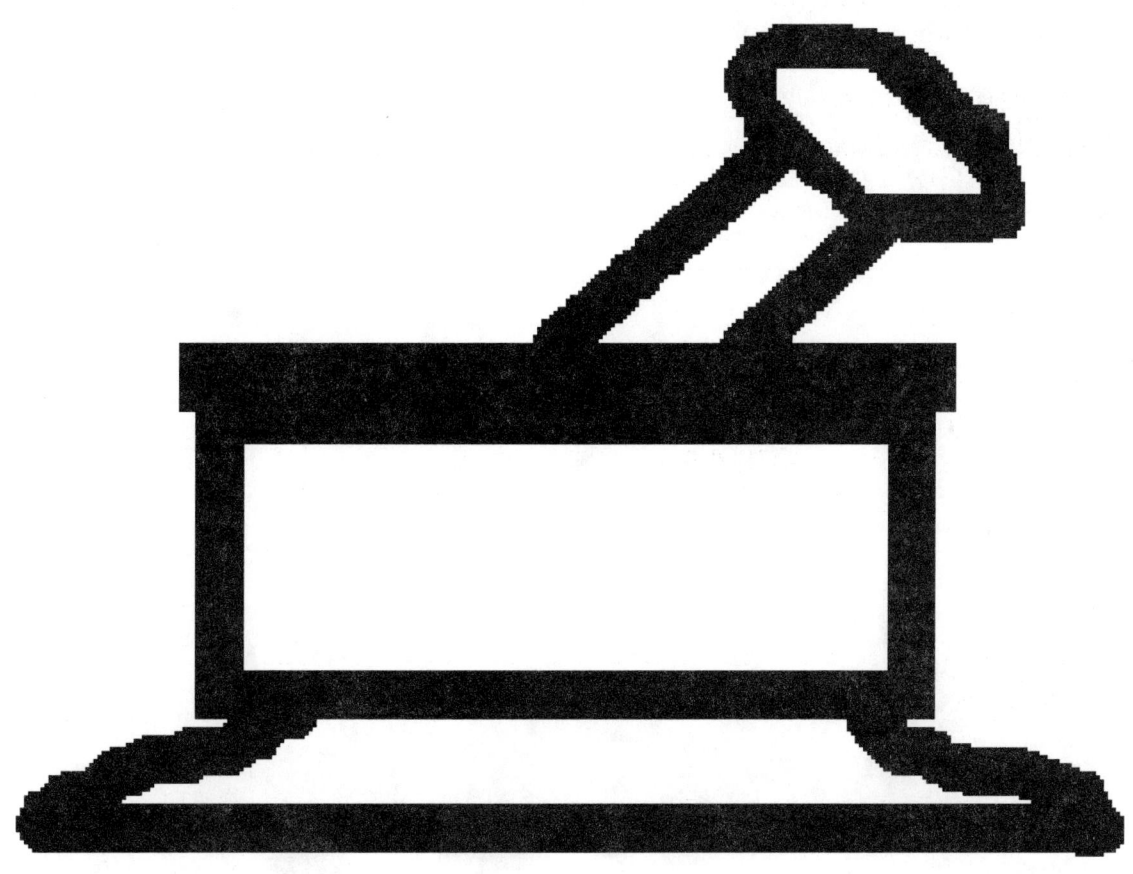

Fraction/Decimal/Ratio/Percent Conversions

Rx Success™ Complete Guide to Medical Math

Fraction/Decimal/Ratio/Percent Conversions

Upon completion of this section, you will be able to convert back and forth between fractions, decimals, ratios and percents. You will see that a fraction is frequently the intermediate between these values.

1. **Decimals and Fractions** – A decimal is readily converted to a fraction by identifying the number of decimal places present. The first place to the right of the decimal is called the "tenths" place. The second place to the right is called the "hundredths" place. The third place to the right is called the "thousandths" place, and so on.

   0.__ TENTHS

   0.0__ HUNDREDTHS

   0.00__ THOUSANDTHS

   If there is only one decimal place (i.e. 0.3 or 0.1) then remove the decimal and place that number over ten. For instance, 0.7 becomes 7/10 (seven tenths). If there are two decimal places (i.e. 0.45 or 0.18) then remove the decimal and place that number over 100. For instance, 0.23 becomes 23/100 (twenty-three hundredths). If there are three decimal places (i.e. 0.375 or 0.623) then remove the decimal and place that number over 1000. For instance, 0.132 becomes 132/1000 (one-hundred thirty-two thousandths).

Decimal	Fraction	Reduced Fraction
0.2	2/10	1/5
0.7	7/10	7/10
0.3	3/10	3/10
0.8	8/10	4/5
0.16	16/100	4/25
0.25	25/100	1/4
0.68	68/100	17/25
0.725	725/1000	29/40
0.419	419/1000	419/1000
0.999	999/1000	999/1000

Rx Success™ Complete Guide to Medical Math

Fractions convert easily to decimals by dividing the top number (the numerator) by the bottom number (the denominator). This is done very simply on a calculator, however, **always make sure to enter the numerator first!**

$$\frac{63 \; \text{Divide}}{90 \; \text{Down!}} = 0.7$$

Fraction	Decimal
5/7	0.71
5/16	0.31
4/5	0.8
7/10	0.7
52/100	0.52
9/18	0.5
65/105	0.62

2. **Fractions and Ratios** – This is perhaps the easiest of the conversions in this section. Fractions and ratios both directly represent relationships between two numbers, whether they are the numerator and denominator of a fraction or the right and left sides of a ratio. To convert a traditional fraction to a ratio, simply rotate the fraction a quarter-turn counter clock-wise and replace the fraction bar with a colon. For the examples listed below, simply replace the fraction bar with a colon.

Fraction	Ratio
5/8	5:8
1/3	1:3
6/7	6:7
1/5	1:5
25/26	25:26

To convert a ratio to a fraction, rotate the ratio a quarter-turn clock-wise (back up to fraction position). For the examples that follow, simply replace the colon with a fraction bar.

Rx Success™ Complete Guide to Medical Math

Ratio	Fraction
7:10	7/10
3:5	3/5
14:17	14/17
1:12	1/12
28:39	28/39

3. **Decimals and Percents** – To convert a **decimal** to a **percent**, multiply the decimal by 100. To convert a **percent** back to a **decimal**, divide the percent by 100. This can be expressed with a simple diagram (see below). It is also common practice to simply move the decimal right or left two places to convert back and forth between percents and decimals. If converting from a **decimal** to a **percent**, move the decimal two places to the right. If converting from a **percent** to a **decimal**, move the decimal two places to the left.

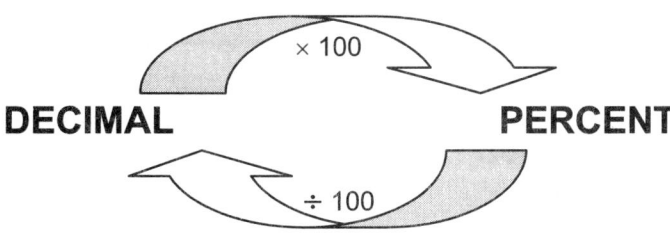

Decimal	Percent
0.16	16%
0.38	38%
0.5	50%
0.75	75%
3.72	372%

4. **Fractions and Percents** – "Percent" is a Latin word that literally means "per 100". So, 17% reads "17 per 100". Which can be written as the fraction 17/100. No matter what the percent, it can be made into a fraction by dropping the percent sign (%) and placing the remaining number over 100. Even if the percent contains a decimal, such as 0.225%, remember **this is *still* a percent!** Regardless of what the number "looks like", if there is a percent sign, **it is a percent!**

Rx Success™ Complete Guide to Medical Math

Percent	Fraction
45%	45/100
3.6%	3.6/100
0.2%	0.2/100
0.75%	0.75/100
75%	75/100
0.09%	0.09/100

Now, continue on to the Sample Problems for this section. The example problems will provide a value as a decimal, fraction, ratio or percent and will then convert that value to another form.

Rx Success™ Complete Guide to Medical Math

Fraction/Decimal/Ratio/Percent Conversions – Sample Problems

Study the following sample problems. Then, continue on to the Tutor Sheets™ and finally the Fraction/Decimal/Ratio/Percent Conversion Homework. Notice that these values are reduced to lowest terms where appropriate. Do not forget to reduce your answers when you complete the homework.

1. Convert 0.725 into a fraction.

To perform this conversion, we must count the decimal places to the right of the decimal. There is a "7" is in the *tenths* position. The "2" is in the *hundredths* position. The "5" is in the *thousandths* position. The one that counts is the position *furthest to the right*, which is the "5". Therefore this fraction is simply

"seven-hundred and twenty-five *thousandths*"

$$\frac{725}{1000}$$

---

2. Convert 90% to a ratio.

   a) As is the case with *every* percent, we must first convert it to a fraction. To do this, simply remove the percent sign and place the remaining number *over* 100.

   90%   becomes $\frac{90}{100}$

   b) The next step it to turn the fraction on its side and replace the fraction bar with a colon. This completes the ratio!

   $\frac{9}{10}$ becomes   9:10

---

3. Convert 1:10,000 to a percent.

   a) As with any ratio, the first step is to convert to a fraction.

Rx Success™ Complete Guide to Medical Math

1:10,000   becomes $\dfrac{1}{10{,}000}$

b) Step two requires us to "divide down" the fraction to convert to a decimal.

1 divided by 10,000 = 0.0001

c) Finally, we must convert the decimal to a percent. To do this, we must multiply the decimal by 100 and add a percent sign.

0.0001 times 100 = 0.01%

Rx Success™ Complete Guide to Medical Math

Fraction/Decimal/Ratio/Percent Conversions - Tutor Sheets™

USE THIS WORKSHEET AS A GUIDE TO HELP YOU SOLVE THE HOMEWORK PROBLEMS!

1. Convert 4/16 into a Ratio, Decimal and Percent

a) Ratio: 4/16 becomes ___:___

b) Decimal: "Divide Down" the fraction.

$\frac{4}{16}$ Divide Down = **0.__ __**

c) Percent: Multiply the Decimal times 100

0.__ __ x 100 = __ __%

2. Convert 0.05% into a Fraction, Ratio and Decimal

a) Fraction: Put the number "over" 100 and drop the percent sign.

0.05% Becomes: $\frac{\_\_.\_\_\_\_}{100}$

b) Ratio: Turn the fraction counter clock-wise.

$\frac{\_\_\_\_}{100}$ Becomes: __.__ __ : __ __ __

c) Decimal: "Divide Down" the fraction.

$\frac{\_\_\_\_}{100}$ Divide Down = **0.__ __ __ __**

Answers to Tutor Sheets™ Calculations

1. a) 4:16 (or ¼)   b) 0.25   c) 25%   2. a) 0.05/100   b) 0.05:100   c) 0.0005

Page - 69

Rx Success™ Complete Guide to Medical Math

Fraction/Decimal/Ratio/Percent Conversions - Homework

Fill in the following table of equivalent measurements. Reduce to lowest terms where appropriate. Follow the example provided.

	Percent	Ratio	Fraction	Decimal
1.	0.01%	1:10,000	1/10,000	0.0001
2.		1:5		
3.			3/96	
4.				0.175
5.				0.4
6.				0.008
7.	15%			
8.			2/15	
9.				0.625
10.			1/12	
11.		1:100		
12.	1.25%			
13.			15/105	
14.			1.5/3	
15.		3:180		
16.		1.75:900		
17.				0.005
18.			7/14.14	
19.	0.0025%			
20.	0.08%			
21.	875%			
22.		1:3000		
23.		115:750		
24.			9/100	
25.			2.5/10	

Rx Success™ Complete Guide to Medical Math

Percent	Ratio	Fraction	Decimal
26.			0.008
27.			0.01
28. 11.5%			
29.	7.5:150.5		
30.			0.35
31.			0.015
32. 12.6%			
33.		10.1/10100	
34.	1:0.05		
35.		250/25	
36.			0.06
37. 90%			
38. 0.225%			
39.	1.5:90		
40.	2:50		
41.		4/5	
42.			0.105
43.		12.5/3.125	
44.	100:5		
45. 8.75%			
46.		1,000/10,000	
47.		50/200,000	
48.			0.00001
49. 10.1%			
50.	12:136		

Rx Success™ Complete Guide to Medical Math

Chapter Seven

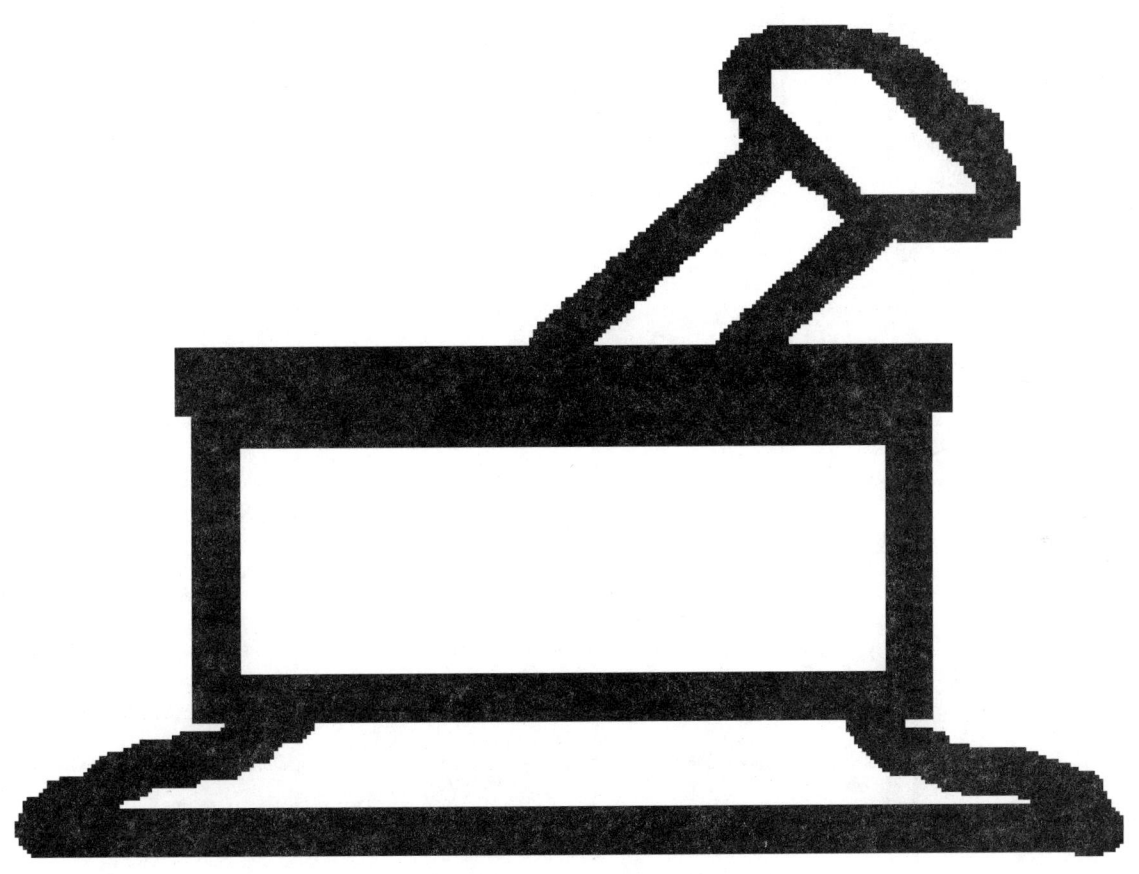

Cross Multiplication

Rx Success™ Complete Guide to Medical Math

Cross Multiplication

Cross multiplication (sometimes referred to as "ratio-proportion") is perhaps the most important skill to learn in medical math. The instinct of most students is to do the simplest of these problems "in their heads" or at best on a calculator without writing anything down. However, these easier problems **must** be done correctly and **written out** in their entirety so that when more difficult problems are encountered, students already have a foundation for these calculations. Also, it must be remembered at all times that patient safety is at stake and patients *deserve* accuracy, even if it takes a bit longer!

The best place to begin looking at cross multiplication is with the formula. Each and every cross multiplication problem will look the same, two fraction bars with an "equals sign" in the middle.

$$\underline{} = \underline{}$$

This setup leaves four places to fill in, two places on the left (top and bottom of the left fraction) and two places on the right (top and bottom of the right fraction). The most important task is to correctly fill in these four fields. These problems should be done in step-wise fashion according to the information below. If you write out every step now, this will help you tremendously when the calculations get more difficult. Additionally, if the problems are set up correctly, you cannot make a mistake! Use the problem below as an example for the following steps.

$$4 \text{ ft} = \underline{} \text{ in}$$

1. **The Code!**
   Every cross multiplication problem has a "code" (aka conversion factor or equivalent) that must be found. For instance, if you were asked how many inches were in four feet, you would probably say 48 inches. Which is correct, but how did you know this? Your mind performed a cross multiplication problem to calculate the correct answer. First, you had to find a known equivalent between the two units in the problem (feet and inches). We will refer to these equivalents as "codes". You knew that the code for this problem was **12 inches = 1 ft**. From that code, you were able to perform a quick cross multiplication problem that told you there were 48 inches in 4 feet. However, when it comes to patient safety, you simply cannot do these calculations in your head.

   Code: 12 in = 1 ft

2. **Code Goes On The Left!**
   Once the code for the problem has been identified, fill it in on the left side of the problem (the top and bottom numbers of the left fraction). The most important thing to remember about this step is to **write the units** when filling in the numbers! This is crucial to the next step. It does not matter which number is

placed on the top or bottom of the left fraction. For instance, you may put "12 inches" on the top and "1 foot" on the bottom (12 inches/1 foot) *or* you may put "1 foot" on the top and "12 inches" on the bottom (1 foot/12 inches). Both are correct and will yield the same answer.

$$\frac{12 \text{ in}}{1 \text{ ft}} = \underline{\qquad} \qquad \text{or} \qquad \frac{1 \text{ ft}}{12 \text{ in}} = \underline{\qquad}$$

3. **Bring the Units Across!**
   The next step is to bring the top and bottom units across. This is very important because you must have the *same units across the top* and the *same units across the bottom*. Looks like this:

$$\frac{12 \text{ in}}{1 \text{ ft}} = \frac{\text{in}}{\text{ft}} \qquad \text{or} \qquad \frac{1 \text{ ft}}{12 \text{ in}} = \frac{\text{ft}}{\text{in}}$$

4. **Fill in the Right Side!**
   Now, you must use information from the problem to fill in the right side of the fraction. Since the units are already labeled, this makes the process easier. The problem told us that we have 4 ft and we are trying to find out how many inches are in those 4 feet. Fill in the "4" on the right side, where it says "ft". Finally, since we are trying to find out how many inches this is, we will fill in an "X" where the "in" units are. Looks like this:

$$\frac{12 \text{ in}}{1 \text{ ft}} = \frac{X \text{ in}}{4 \text{ ft}} \qquad \text{or} \qquad \frac{1 \text{ ft}}{12 \text{ in}} = \frac{4 \text{ in}}{X \text{ in}}$$

5. **Cross Multiplication!**
   For the next step we will use this setup: 12 in/1 ft = X in/4 ft. Cross up from the bottom right to the top left, multiply the two numbers together (4 times 12) and write the answer below (48). Do not bring the units along, just write the number below the problem. Then, bring down the "equals sign" to the second line, like this:

$$\frac{12 \text{ in}}{1 \text{ ft}} = \frac{X \text{ in}}{4 \text{ ft}}$$

$$48 \quad =$$

Then, cross from the bottom left to the top right (1 times X = X) and write the answer below, like this:

$$\frac{12 \text{ in}}{1 \text{ ft}} = \frac{X \text{ in}}{4 \text{ ft}}$$

$$48 \quad = \quad X$$

Rx Success™ Complete Guide to Medical Math

The object of a cross multiplication problem is to find out what "X" is, so this problem is done!

Study the Sample Problems that follow and then complete the Cross Multiplication Tutor Sheets™ and Homework at the end of this chapter.

Rx Success™ Complete Guide to Medical Math

Cross Multiplication – Sample Problems

Study the following sample problems and then move on to complete the Cross Multiplication Tutor Sheets™ and Homework at the end of this chapter.

1. **62 min = _____ sec**

    $$\frac{X\ sec}{62\ min} = \frac{60\ sec}{1\ min}$$

    $$X = 3720\ secs$$

    a) **Find the Code** – The code between seconds and minutes is

    60 sec = 1 min

    b) **Code Goes on the Left** – Fill in the code on the left side of the problem. Remember, you may place either "60 sec" *or* "1 min" on top, it does not matter which.

    $$\frac{60\ sec}{1\ min} = _____$$

    c) **Bring the Units Across** – Make sure your units match across the top and bottom. Bring "sec" across the top and "min" across the bottom.

    $$\frac{60\ sec}{1\ min} = \frac{\_\_\_\_\_\ sec}{min}$$

    d) **Fill in the Right Side** – Look back at the original question for the information necessary to fill in the remaining two spaces in the cross multiplication problem.

    $$\frac{60\ sec}{1\ min} = \frac{X\ sec}{62\ min}$$

    e) **Cross Multiply** – Cross multiply both sides (follow the arrows) and write the resulting numbers below. Do not forget to bring the "equals sign" down.

    $$\frac{60\ sec}{1\ min} = \frac{X\ sec}{62\ min}$$

    $$3720 = X$$

    The final answer is **3720 sec.**

Rx Success™ Complete Guide to Medical Math

2. 39 in = _____ ft

   a) **Find the Code** – The code between in and ft is

   $$\frac{X \text{ ft}}{39 \text{ in}} = \frac{1 \text{ ft}}{12 \text{ in}}$$

   $$12X = 39$$
   $$X = 3.25 \text{ ft}$$

   12 in = 1 ft

   b) **Code Goes on the Left** – Fill in the code on the left side of the problem. Remember, you may place either the 12 in *or* the 1 ft on top, it does not matter which.

   $$\frac{12 \text{ in}}{1 \text{ ft}} = \underline{\qquad}$$

   c) **Bring the Units Across** – Make sure your units match across the top and bottom. Bring "in" across the top and "ft" across the bottom.

   $$\frac{12 \text{ in}}{1 \text{ ft}} = \frac{\text{in}}{\text{ft}}$$

   d) **Fill in the Right Side** – Look back at the original question for the information necessary to fill in the remaining two spaces in the cross multiplication problem.

   $$\frac{12 \text{ in}}{1 \text{ ft}} = \frac{39 \text{ in}}{X \text{ ft}}$$

   e) **Cross Multiply** – Cross multiply both sides (follow the arrows) and write the resulting numbers below. Do not forget to bring the "equals sign" down.

   $$\frac{12 \text{ in}}{1 \text{ ft}} \diagdown\!\!\!\!\diagup \frac{39 \text{ in}}{X \text{ ft}}$$

   $$39 = 12X$$

   f) **Get "X" By Itself** – This time, we had to multiply X by a number other than "1". This forces us to get rid of the number in front of the X. In this case, the number is "12". To get rid of the 12, put both sides of the equation "over" 12. This will get X by itself because the 12's will cancel each other out. This leaves us with a fraction for an answer (X = 39/12). Simply "divide down" the fraction and get a decimal (39 divided by 12 = 3.25). Looks like this:

$$\frac{39}{12} = \frac{12X}{12}$$

$$\frac{39}{12} = X$$

$$3.25 = X$$

The final answer is **3.25 ft.**

Rx Success™ Complete Guide to Medical Math

Cross Multiplication - *Tutor Sheets*™

USE THIS WORKSHEET AS A GUIDE TO HELP YOU SOLVE THE HOMEWORK PROBLEMS!

---

1. 154 ft = _____ in   Code: 1 ft = 12 in

$$\frac{12 \text{ in}}{1 \text{ ft}} = \frac{X \text{ in}}{154 \text{ ft}}$$

$$x = 1848 \text{ in}$$

$$\frac{12 \text{ in}}{1 \text{ ft}} \diagup\!\!\!= \frac{X \text{ in}}{154 \text{ ft}}$$

X = _____

$$\frac{X \text{ in}}{154 \text{ ft}} = \frac{12 \text{ in}}{1 \text{ ft}}$$

$$x = 1848 \text{ in}$$

---

2. 68 min = _____ sec   Code: 60 sec = 1 min

$$\frac{60 \text{ sec}}{1 \text{ min}} \diagup\!\!\!= \frac{X \text{ sec}}{68 \text{ min}}$$

X = 4080 sec

$$\frac{X \text{ sec}}{68 \text{ min}} = \frac{60 \text{ sec}}{1 \text{ min}}$$

$$X = 4080 \text{ secs}$$

---

3. 18 ft = _____ yd   Code: 3 ft = 1 yd

$$\frac{3 \text{ ft}}{1 \text{ yd}} \diagup\!\!\!= \frac{18 \text{ ft}}{X \text{ yd}}$$

$$\frac{3X \text{ yd}}{3 \text{ ft}} = \frac{18 \text{ ft}}{3 \text{ ft}}$$

$$\frac{12 \text{ in}}{1 \text{ ft}} = \frac{X \text{ in}}{3 \text{ ft}} \qquad 36 = X$$

X = 6 yd

$$\frac{X \text{ yd}}{18 \text{ ft}} = \frac{1 \text{ yd}}{3 \text{ ft}}$$

$$3x = 18$$
$$x = 6 \text{ yd}$$

---

4. 90 in = _____ yd   Code: 36 in = 1 yd

$$\frac{36 \text{ in}}{1 \text{ yd}} = \frac{90 \text{ in}}{X \text{ yd}} \qquad 90 = 36x$$

$$x = 2.5 \text{ yds}$$

$$\frac{X \text{ yd}}{90 \text{ in}} = \frac{1 \text{ yd}}{36 \text{ in}}$$

$$36x = 90$$
$$x = 2.5 \text{ yd}$$

Rx Success™ Complete Guide to Medical Math

_____ ⤫ _____

_____ = _____

X = _____

---

5. 62 in = _____ ft   Code: _____ = _____

_____ ⤫ _____

$$\frac{x \text{ ft}}{62 \text{ in}} = \frac{1 \text{ ft}}{12 \text{ in}}$$

_____ = _____

$$12x = 62$$
$$x = 5.17 \text{ ft}$$

X = _____

---

6. 264 min = _____ hr   Code: _____ = _____

_____ ⤫ _____

$$\frac{x \text{ hr}}{264 \text{ min}} = \frac{1 \text{ hr}}{60 \text{ min}}$$

_____ = _____

$$60x = 264$$
$$x = 4.4 \text{ hrs}$$

X = _____

Rx Success™ Complete Guide to Medical Math

7. 4800 in = _____ ft   Code: _____ = _____

_____ = _____

$$\frac{x \text{ ft}}{4800 \text{ in}} = \frac{1 \text{ ft}}{12 \text{ in}}$$

$$12x = 4800$$

$$x = 400 \text{ ft}$$

X = _____

---

8. 0.75 yd = _____ in   Code: _____ = _____

$$\frac{x \text{ ft}}{0.75 \text{ yd}} = \frac{3 \text{ ft}}{1 \text{ yd}}$$

$$x = 2.25 \text{ ft}$$

$$\frac{x \text{ in}}{2.25 \text{ ft}} = \frac{12 \text{ in}}{1 \text{ ft}}$$

X = _____

$$x = 27 \text{ in}$$

---

9. 960 sec = _____ hr   Code: _____ = _____

_____ = _____

$$\frac{x \text{ min}}{960 \text{ sec}} = \frac{1 \text{ min}}{60 \text{ sec}}$$

$$60x = 960$$

$$x = 16 \text{ min}$$

X = _____

$$\frac{x \text{ hr}}{16 \text{ min}} = \frac{1 \text{ hr}}{60 \text{ min}}$$

$$60x = 16$$

$$x = 0.27 \text{ hr}$$

Rx Success™ Complete Guide to Medical Math

10. 46,260 in = _____ yd   Code: _____ = _____

$$\frac{X \text{ yd}}{46260 \text{ in}} = \frac{1 \text{ yd}}{36 \text{ in}}$$

$$36 X = 46260$$

$$X = 1285 \text{ yd}$$

_____ = _____

X = _____

Answers to Tutor Sheets™ Calculations

1) 1848 in   2) 4080 sec   3) 6 yd   4) 2.5 yd   5) 5.17 ft   6) 4.4 hr   7) 400 ft   8) 27 in
9) 0.27 hr   10) 1285 yd

Rx Success™ Complete Guide to Medical Math
Cross Multiplication - Homework

Use cross multiplication to calculate the following problems.

1. 25 min = _____ sec

    $\dfrac{60 \text{ sec}}{1 \text{ min}} = \dfrac{x \text{ sec}}{25 \text{ min}}$ $1500 = x$

2. 116 min = _____ sec

    $\dfrac{60 \text{ sec}}{1 \text{ min}} = \dfrac{x \text{ sec}}{116 \text{ min}}$ $6960 = x$

3. 12.6 ft = _____ in

    $\dfrac{12 \text{ in}}{1 \text{ ft}} = \dfrac{x \text{ in}}{12.6 \text{ ft}}$ $x = 151.2 \text{ in}$

4. 0.75 ft = _____ in

    $\dfrac{12 \text{ in}}{1 \text{ ft}} = \dfrac{x \text{ in}}{0.75 \text{ ft}}$ $x = 9 \text{ in}$

5. 8.5 hr = _____ min

    $\dfrac{60 \text{ min}}{1 \text{ hr}} = \dfrac{x \text{ min}}{8.5 \text{ hr}}$ $x = 510 \text{ min}$

6. 0.5 yd = _____ ft

    $\dfrac{3 \text{ ft}}{1 \text{ yd}} = \dfrac{x \text{ ft}}{0.5 \text{ yd}}$ $x = 1.5 \text{ ft}$

7. 360 sec = _____ min

    $\dfrac{60 \text{ sec}}{1 \text{ min}} = \dfrac{360 \text{ sec}}{x \text{ min}}$ $360 = 60x$ $x = 6 \text{ min}$

Rx Success™ Complete Guide to Medical Math

8. 3600 sec = __1__ hr

$\dfrac{60 \text{ sec}}{1 \text{ min}} = \dfrac{x \text{ sec}}{60 \text{ min}}$

3600 sec = x

$\dfrac{60 \text{ sec}}{1 \text{ min}}$

9. 72 sec = _____ min

$\dfrac{60 \text{ sec}}{1 \text{ min}} = \dfrac{72 \text{ sec}}{x \text{ min}}$ 72 = 60x   x = 1.2 min

10. 156 feet = _____ yd

$\dfrac{3 f}{1 \text{ yd}} = \dfrac{156 \text{ ft}}{x \text{ yd}}$ 156 = 3x   x = 52 yd

11. 1200 sec = _____ min

$\dfrac{60 \text{ sec}}{1 \text{ min}} = \dfrac{1200 \text{ sec}}{x \text{ min}}$ 60x = 1200   x = 20 min

12. 600 in = _____ feet

$\dfrac{12 \text{ in}}{1 \text{ ft}} = \dfrac{600 \text{ in}}{x \text{ ft}}$ 12x = 600   x = 50 ft

13. 72,000 in = _____ yd

$\dfrac{36 \text{ in}}{1 \text{ yd}} = \dfrac{72000 \text{ in}}{x \text{ yd}}$ 36x = 72000   x = 2000 yd

14. 186 sec = _____ min

$\dfrac{60 \text{ sec}}{1 \text{ min}} = \dfrac{186 \text{ sec}}{x \text{ min}}$ 60x = 186   x = 3.1 min

15. 91.5 feet = _____ yd

$\dfrac{3 \text{ ft}}{1 \text{ yd}} = \dfrac{91.5 \text{ ft}}{x \text{ yd}}$ 3x = 91.5   x = 30.5 yd

Rx Success™ Complete Guide to Medical Math

16. 81 yd = _____ in $\dfrac{36 \text{ in}}{1 \text{ yd}} = \dfrac{x \text{ in}}{81 \text{ yd}}$ $x = 2916 \text{ in}$

17. 214 in = _____ yd $\dfrac{36 \text{ in}}{1 \text{ yd}} = \dfrac{214 \text{ in}}{x \text{ yd}}$ $36x = 214$ $x = 5.94 \text{ yd}$

18. 8200 sec = _____ hr $\dfrac{3600 \text{ sec}}{1 \text{ hr}} = \dfrac{8200 \text{ sec}}{x \text{ hr}}$ $3600x = 8200$ $x = 2.28$

19. 9.3 yd = _____ in $\dfrac{36 \text{ in}}{1 \text{ yd}} = \dfrac{x \text{ in}}{9.3 \text{ yd}}$ $x = 334.8 \text{ in}$

20. 17 hr = _____ sec $\dfrac{3600 \text{ sec}}{1 \text{ hr}} = \dfrac{x \text{ sec}}{17 \text{ hr}}$ $x = 61200 \text{ sec}$

Rx Success™ Complete Guide to Medical Math

Chapter Eight

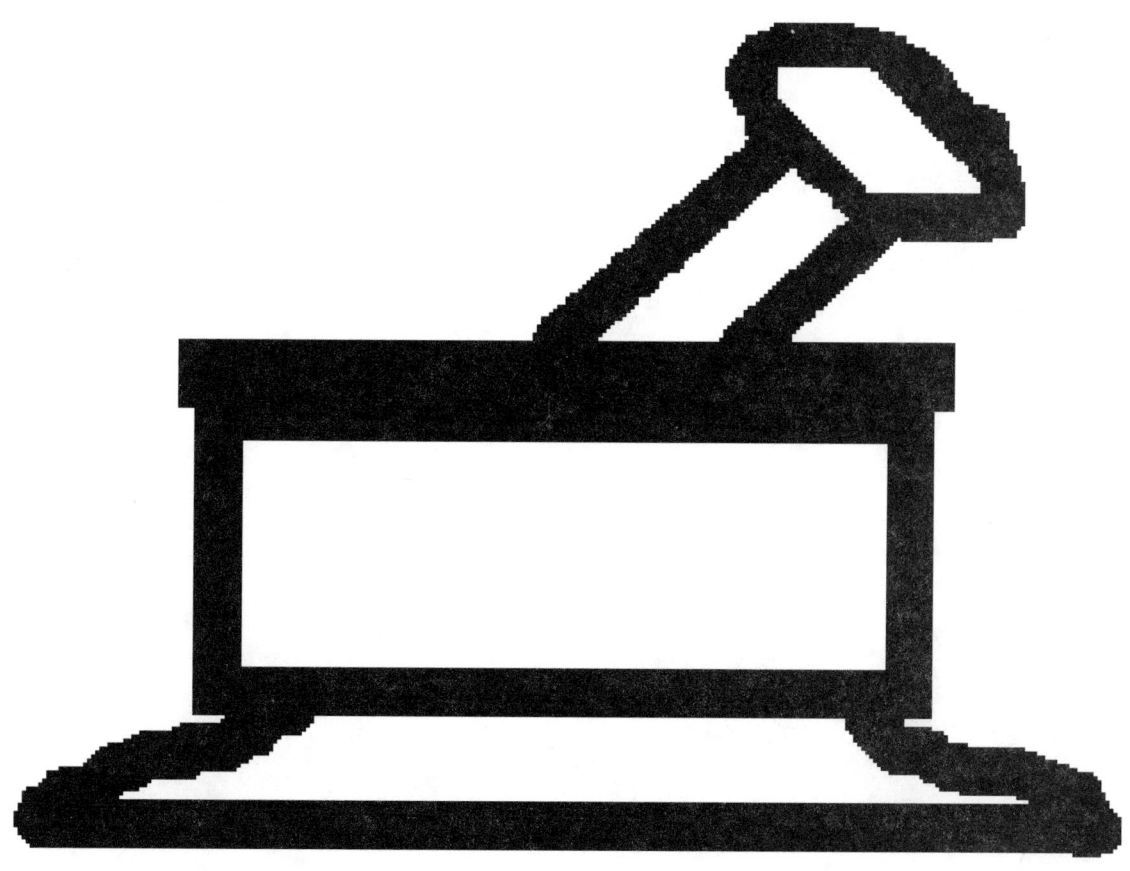

Apothecary, Household and Metric Conversions

Rx Success™ Complete Guide to Medical Math

Apothecary, Household and Metric Conversions

The conversions in this section are calculated like any other cross multiplication problem. First find the code, then perform each of the steps in order. You may not be familiar with all of the equivalents used for these conversions, however, **many of these equivalents must be memorized! Here are some that must be committed to memory.**

1cc = 1mL

60mg	=		1 grain (gr)
★ 5mL	=		1 teaspoon ★
★ 15mL	=	3 teaspoons =	1 tablespoon ★
★ 30mL	=		1 ounce ★
4mL	=		1 dram
1L	=	1 quart =	2 pints
★ 480mL	=		1 pint

The above are approximate equivalents but they are accepted by the industry and are appropriate to use for calculations.

The ability to convert back and forth between household, apothecary and metric systems is an absolute necessity. Often, physicians write medication orders in units that are different than those units on the label of the actual medication. For instance, suppose you receive the following order...

Order: Patient A is to receive 1.2 g of magnesium sulfate.

Upon retrieving the bottle of magnesium sulfate, here is what you read on the medication label...

Magnesium Sulfate: 500 mg/ml

Notice that the physician's order is in strength units of **"grams"** and the strength units on the actual drug is **"milligrams"**. This inconsistency makes it necessary to convert *either* the order into milligrams *or* the drug strength into grams. Either way, the end result is the same: Both strengths are measured in the same strength units! There are also many other circumstances where it is necessary to perform a conversion. Suppose a child is to receive the following amount of a liquid drug...

Order: 10 mls of medication

However, the child's mother does not have a device for accurately measuring milliliters. She does have a device for accurately measuring teaspoons. This makes it necessary for you to convert "10 mls" into "teaspoons".

Rx Success™ Complete Guide to Medical Math

There are many other applications for these skills. For some calculations, you will also need to incorporate fraction/decimal/ratio/percent conversions! It is important to remember that the majority of these calculations are simply cross multiplication problems. Therefore it is extremely important to perfect this skill (see Chapter 7) before moving on to the calculations that follow in this chapter. These types of problems may seem difficult initially, however, the more you practice, the more confident you will become.

Review the Sample Problems that follow and then fill in the Tutor Sheets™. This will prepare you to complete the homework at the end of this section.

Rx Success™ Complete Guide to Medical Math

Apothecary, Household and Metric Conversions – Sample Problems

Study the following sample problems and then move on to complete the Cross Multiplication Tutor Sheets™ and Homework at the end of this chapter. Remember to keep the Conversion Factor Quickview handy as you may need to refer back to it to complete these problems.

1. 23 oz = _____ ml

    $$\frac{X \text{ ml}}{23 \text{ oz}} = \frac{30 \text{ ml}}{1 \text{ oz}} \quad X = 690 \text{ ml}$$

   a) **Find the Code** – The code between ml and oz is that 30 ml = 1 oz

      Code: 30 ml = 1 oz

   b) **Code Goes on the Left** – Fill in the code on the left side of the problem. Remember, you may place either the 30 ml or the 1 oz on top, it does not matter which.

      $$\frac{30 \text{ ml}}{1 \text{ oz}} = \underline{\qquad}$$

   c) **Bring the Units Across** – Bring "ml" across the top and "oz" across the bottom.

      $$\frac{30 \text{ ml}}{1 \text{ oz}} = \frac{\underline{\qquad} \text{ ml}}{\text{oz}}$$

   d) **Fill in the Right Side** – Look back at the original question for the information necessary to fill in the remaining two spaces in the cross multiplication problem.

      $$\frac{30 \text{ ml}}{1 \text{ oz}} = \frac{X \text{ ml}}{23 \text{ oz}}$$

   e) **Cross Multiply** – Cross multiply both sides (follow the arrows) and write the resulting numbers below. Do not forget to bring the "equals sign" down.

Rx Success™ Complete Guide to Medical Math

$$\frac{30 \text{ ml}}{1 \text{ oz}} \diagdown \diagup \frac{X \text{ ml}}{23 \text{ oz}}$$

690 = X

The final answer is **690 mls.**

---

2.   **615 ml = _____ T** $\frac{XT}{615mL} = \frac{1T}{15mL}$ $15x = 615$
   $x = 41 T$

a) **Find the Code** – The code between ml and T is that 15 ml = 1 T

   Code: 15 ml = 1 T

b) **Code Goes on the Left** – Fill in the code on the left side of the problem. Remember, you may place either the 15 ml or the 1 T on top, it does not matter which.

$$\frac{15 \text{ ml}}{1 \text{ T}} = \underline{\qquad}$$

c) **Bring the Units Across** – Bring "ml" across the top and "T" across the bottom.

$$\frac{15 \text{ ml}}{1 \text{ T}} = \frac{\text{ml}}{\text{T}}$$

d) **Fill in the Right Side** – Look back at the original question for the information necessary to fill in the remaining two spaces in the cross multiplication.

$$\frac{15 \text{ ml}}{1 \text{ T}} = \frac{615 \text{ ml}}{X \text{ T}}$$

e) **Cross Multiply** – Cross multiply both sides (follow the arrows) and write the resulting numbers below. Do not forget to bring the "equals sign" down.

Rx Success™ Complete Guide to Medical Math

$$\frac{15 \text{ ml}}{1 \text{ T}} \underset{\searrow}{\overset{\nearrow}{=}} \frac{615 \text{ ml}}{X \text{ T}}$$

15X = 615

f) **Get "X" By Itself** – This time, we had to multiply X by a number other than "1". This forces us to get rid of the number in front of the X. In this case, the number is "15". To get rid of the 15, put both sides of the equation "over" 15. This will get X by itself because the 15's will cancel each other. This leaves us with a fraction for an answer (X = 615/15). Simply "divide down" the fraction and get a decimal (615 divided by 15 = 41). Looks like this:

$$15X = 615$$

$$\frac{\cancel{15} \, X}{\cancel{15}} = \frac{615}{15}$$

$$X = 41$$

---

3.   2.5 gr = _____ mg   Code: 60 mg = 1 gr

$\frac{X \, mg}{2.5 \, gr} = \frac{60 \, mg}{1 \, gr}$ x = 150 mg

$$\frac{60 \text{ mg}}{1 \text{ gr}} \underset{\searrow}{\overset{\nearrow}{=}} \frac{X \text{ mg}}{2.5 \text{ gr}}$$

X = 150 mg

---

4.   4 T = _____ ml   Code: 15 ml = 1 T

$\frac{X \, mL}{4T} = \frac{15 \, mL}{1T}$ x = 60 mL

$$\frac{15 \text{ ml}}{1 \text{ T}} \underset{\searrow}{\overset{\nearrow}{=}} \frac{X \text{ ml}}{4 \text{ T}}$$

X = 60 ml

Rx Success™ Complete Guide to Medical Math

5. **2.5 pt = _____ ml**   Code: 480 ml = 1 pt

$$\frac{X\ ml}{2.5\ pt} = \frac{480\ ml}{1\ pt}$$
$$x = 1200\ ml$$

$$\frac{480\ ml}{1\ pt} \diagdown\!\!\!\!\!= \frac{X\ ml}{2.5\ pt}$$

X = 1200 ml

---

6. **36 ml = _____ dr**   Code: 4 ml = 1 dr

$$\frac{X\ dr}{36\ ml} = \frac{1\ dr}{4\ ml}$$
$$4x = 36$$
$$x = 9\ dr$$

$$\frac{4\ ml}{1\ dr} \diagdown\!\!\!\!\!= \frac{36\ ml}{X\ dr}$$

$$4X = 36$$

X = 9 dr

---

7. **26 dr = _____ oz**   a) Code: 4 ml = 1 dr
            b) Code: 30 ml = 1 oz

a. $\frac{4\ ml}{1\ dr} \diagdown\!\!\!\!\!= \frac{X\ ml}{26\ dr}$ ⇒   X = 104 ml

$$\frac{X\ mL}{26\ dr} = \frac{4\ mL}{1\ dr}$$
$$X = 104\ mL$$

b. $\frac{30\ ml}{1\ oz} \diagdown\!\!\!\!\!= \frac{104\ ml}{X\ oz}$ ⇒ $X = \frac{104}{30}$

$$\frac{X\ oz}{104\ mL} = \frac{1\ oz}{30\ mL}$$
$$30X = 104$$
$$X = 3.47\ oz$$

X = 3.47 oz

Rx Success™ Complete Guide to Medical Math

Apothecary, Household and Metric Conversions - Tutor Sheets™

USE THIS WORKSHEET AS A GUIDE TO HELP YOU SOLVE THE HOMEWORK PROBLEMS!

---

1. 45 ml = _____ oz   Code: 30 ml = 1 oz

$$\frac{X \, oz}{45 \, mL} = \frac{1 \, oz}{30 \, mL}$$

$30x = 45$

$x = 1.5 \, oz$

$$\frac{30 \, ml}{1 \, oz} \underset{\times}{=} \frac{45 \, ml}{X \, oz}$$

$$\frac{30 X}{30} = \frac{45}{30}$$

X = _____

---

2. 450 gr = _____ mg   Code: _____ = _____

$$\frac{X \, mg}{450 \, gr} = \frac{60 \, mg}{1 \, gr}$$

$x = 27000 \, mg$

X = _____

---

3. 2040 ml = _____ pt   Code: _____ = _____

$$\frac{X \, pt}{2040 \, mL} = \frac{1 \, pt}{480 \, mL}$$

$480x = 2040$

$x = 4.25 \, pt$

_____ = _____

X = _____

---

4. 105 ml = _____ T $\frac{X \, T}{105 \, mL} = \frac{1 \, T}{15 \, mL}$ Code: _____ = _____

$15x = 105$

$x = 7 \, T$

Rx Success™ Complete Guide to Medical Math

_____ = _____

X = _____

---

5. 8.6 pt = _____ ml

$$\frac{x\ mL}{8.6\ pt} = \frac{480\ mL}{1\ pt}$$

x = 4128 mL

Code: _____ = _____

X = _____

---

6. 80.5 dr = _____ ml

$$\frac{x\ mL}{80.5\ dr} = \frac{4\ mL}{1\ dr}$$

x = 322 mL

Code: _____ = _____

X = _____

---

7. 275 ml = _____ t

$$\frac{x\ t}{275\ mL} = \frac{1\ t}{5\ mL}$$

5x = 275

x = 55 t

Code: _____ = _____

_____ = _____

X = _____

Rx Success™ Complete Guide to Medical Math

8. 1480 ml = _____ pt   Code: _____ = _____

$$\frac{X \text{ pt}}{1480 \text{ mL}} = \frac{1 \text{ pt}}{480 \text{ mL}}$$

$480 x = 1480$

$x = 3.08 \text{ pt}$

_____ = _____

X = _____

---

9. 2.5 pt = _____ dr

Step One: Since we do not have a direct code (equivalent) between pints and drams, we must perform this conversion in two steps. First, we will convert 2.5 pt into ml. Finally, we will convert ml into dr.   Code: _____ pt = _____ ml

$$\frac{X \text{ mL}}{2.5 \text{ pt}} = \frac{480 \text{ mL}}{1 \text{ pt}}$$

$X = 1200 \text{ mL}$

$$\frac{X \text{ dr}}{1200 \text{ mL}} = \frac{1 \text{ dr}}{4 \text{ mL}}$$

$4x = 1200 \quad x = 300 \text{ dr}$

X = _____ ml

Step Two: Convert ml to dr   Code: _____ ml = _____ dr

_____ = _____

X = _____ dr

---

10. 85 T = _____ pt

$$\frac{X \text{ mL}}{85 \text{ T}} = \frac{15 \text{ mL}}{1 \text{ T}}$$

Step One: Convert T to ml $X = 1275 \text{ mL}$ Code: _____ T = _____ ml

$$\frac{X \text{ pt}}{1275 \text{ mL}} = \frac{1 \text{ pt}}{480 \text{ mL}} \quad 480 x = 1275 \quad x = 2.66 \text{ pt}$$

Rx Success™ Complete Guide to Medical Math

X = _____ ml

Step Two: Convert ml to pt   Code: _____ ml = _____ pt

_____ = _____

X = _____ pt

Answers to Tutor Sheets™ Calculations
1) 1.5 oz   2) 27,000 mg   3) 4.25 pt   4) 7 T   5) 4128 ml   6) 322 ml   7) 55 t   8) 3.08 pt   9) 300 dr   10) 2.66 pt

Rx Success™ Complete Guide to Medical Math

Apothecary, Household and Metric Conversions - Homework

Use cross multiplication to calculate the following problems.

1. 16 qt = ____32____ pt

    $$\frac{X\,pt}{16\,qt} = \frac{2\,pt}{1\,qt} \qquad x = 32\,pt$$

2. 720 mg = ____12____ gr

    $$\frac{X\,gr}{720\,mg} = \frac{1\,gr}{60\,mg} \qquad \begin{array}{l} 60x = 720 \\ x = 12\,gr \end{array}$$

3. 100 ml = ____20____ t

    $$\frac{X\,t}{100\,mL} = \frac{1\,t}{5\,mL} \qquad \begin{array}{l} 5x = 100 \\ x = 20\,t \end{array}$$

4. 6.5 T = ____97.5____ ml

    $$\frac{X\,mL}{6.5\,T} = \frac{15\,mL}{1\,T} \qquad x = 97.5\,mL$$

5. 112 cc = ____28____ dr

    $$\frac{4\,cc}{1\,dr} = \frac{112\,cc}{X\,dr} \qquad \begin{array}{l} 4x = 112 \\ x = 28\,dr \end{array}$$

6. 15.6 gr = ____936____ mg

    $$\frac{X\,mg}{15.6\,gr} = \frac{60\,mg}{1\,gr} \qquad x = 936\,mg$$

7. 2.75 oz = ____82.5____ ml

    $$\frac{X\,mL}{2.75\,oz} = \frac{30\,mL}{1\,oz} \qquad x = 82.5\,mL$$

8. 45 mg = ____0.75____ gr

    $$\frac{X\,gr}{45\,mg} = \frac{1\,gr}{60\,mg} \qquad \begin{array}{l} 60x = 45 \\ x = 0.75\,gr \end{array}$$

9. 100.5 dr = ____402____ ml

    $$\frac{X\,mL}{100.5\,dr} = \frac{4\,mL}{1\,dr} \qquad x = 402\,mL$$

Rx Success™ Complete Guide to Medical Math

10. 7.5 gr = __450__ mg

$$\frac{x\,mg}{7.5\,gr} = \frac{60\,mg}{1\,gr} \quad x = 450\,mg$$

11. 240 cc = __60__ dr

$$\frac{x\,dr}{240\,cc} = \frac{1\,dr}{4\,cc} \quad \begin{array}{l} 4x = 240 \\ x = 60\,dr \end{array}$$

12. 0.5 ml = __0.125__ dr

$$\frac{x\,dr}{0.5\,mL} = \frac{1\,dr}{4\,mL} \quad \begin{array}{l} 4x = 0.5 \\ x = 0.125\,dr \end{array}$$

13. 3.5 oz = __105__ ml

$$\frac{30\,mL}{1\,oz} = \frac{x\,mL}{3.5\,oz} \quad x = 105\,ml$$

14. 30 T = __450__ ml

$$\frac{x\,mL}{30\,T} = \frac{15\,mL}{1\,T} \quad x = 450\,mL$$

15. 56 T = __28 oz__ oz

$$\frac{x\,oz}{15\,mL} = \frac{1\,oz}{30\,mL} \quad \begin{array}{l} 30x = 15 \\ x = 0.5\,oz \end{array} \quad \frac{x\,oz}{56\,T} = \frac{0.5\,oz}{1\,T} \quad x = 28\,oz$$

16. 1875 mg = __31.25__ gr

$$\frac{x\,gr}{1875\,mg} = \frac{1\,gr}{60\,mg} \quad \begin{array}{l} 60x = 1875 \\ x = 31.25\,gr \end{array}$$

17. 64 t = __320__ ml

$$\frac{x\,mL}{64\,t} = \frac{5\,mL}{1\,t} \quad x = 320\,mL$$

18. 120 oz = __3600__ ml

$$\frac{x\,mL}{120\,oz} = \frac{30\,mL}{1\,oz} \quad x = 3600\,mL$$

19. 1920 ml = __4__ pt

$$\frac{x\,pt}{1920\,mL} = \frac{1\,pt}{480\,mL} \quad \begin{array}{l} 480x = 1920 \\ x = 4\,pt \end{array}$$

Rx Success™ Complete Guide to Medical Math

20. 2.4 L = __2.4__ qt

The following problems involve 2-step conversions (you may be able to do them in one step if you remember the correct conversion factor!).

21. 27 pt = __432__ oz

$$\frac{X\,oz}{480\,mL} = \frac{1\,oz}{30\,mL} \quad 30x=480 \quad x=16\,oz \quad \boxed{so\ 1\,pt=16\,oz} \quad \frac{X\,oz}{27\,pt} = \frac{16\,oz}{1\,pt} \quad X=432\,oz$$

22. 7.5 gr = __0.45__ g

$$\frac{X\,g}{7.5\,gr} = \frac{0.06\,g}{1\,gr} \quad x=0.45\,g \qquad \frac{X\,g}{60\,mg} = \frac{1\,g}{1000\,mg} \quad 1000x=60 \quad X=0.06\,g \quad \boxed{1\,gr=0.06\,g}$$

23. 21 pt = __2520__ dr

$$\frac{X\,dr}{480\,mL} = \frac{1\,dr}{4\,mL} \quad 4x=480 \quad x=120\,dr \quad \boxed{so\ 120\,dr=1\,pt} \quad \frac{X\,dr}{21\,pt} = \frac{120\,dr}{1\,pt} \quad X=2520\,dr$$

24. 15 dr = __2__ oz

$$\frac{X\,oz}{4\,mL} = \frac{1\,oz}{30\,mL} \quad 30x=4 \quad x=0.133\,oz \quad \boxed{so\ 1\,dr=0.133\,oz} \quad \frac{X\,oz}{15\,dr} = \frac{0.133\,oz}{1\,dr} \quad X=1.995\,oz$$

25. 0.5 T = __0.25__ oz

$$\frac{2\,T}{1\,oz} = \frac{0.5\,T}{X\,oz} \quad 2x=0.5\,oz \quad x=0.25$$

26. 2.5 oz = __18.8__ dr

$$\frac{X\,dr}{2.5\,oz} = \frac{1\,dr}{0.133\,oz} \quad 0.133x=2.5 \quad x=18.8\,dr \qquad \frac{X\,dr}{30\,mL} = \frac{1\,dr}{4\,mL} \quad 4x=30 \quad x=7.5\,dr \quad \boxed{7.5\,dr=1\,oz}$$

27. 220 t = __2.3__ pt

$$\frac{X\,pt}{5\,mL} = \frac{1\,pt}{480\,mL} \quad 480x=5 \quad x=0.0104\,pt \quad \boxed{1\,t=0.0104\,pt} \quad \frac{X\,pt}{220\,t} = \frac{0.0104\,pt}{1\,t} \quad X=2.3\,pt$$

28. 96 oz = __6__ pt

$$\frac{X\,pt}{96\,oz} = \frac{1\,pt}{16\,oz} \quad 16x=96 \quad x=6\,pt$$

Rx Success™ Complete Guide to Medical Math

29. 0.5 pt = __48.08__ t

30. 0.5 oz = __1__ T

31. 60 dr = __8__ oz

32. 86 T = __2.69__ pt

33. 150 g = __2500.5__ gr

34. 7 gr = __420__ mg

35. 104 T = __390__ dr

36. 20.5 oz = __1.28__ pt

37. 16.8 oz = __100.8__ t

38. 120 t = __1.25__ pt

Rx Success™ Complete Guide to Medical Math

39. 1.5 qt = __50__ oz

$$\frac{X\,oz}{1000\,mL} = \frac{1\,oz}{30\,mL} \quad 30x = 1000 \quad x = 33.33\,oz \quad \boxed{so\ 1\,qt = 33.33\,oz}$$

$$\frac{X\,oz}{1.5\,qt} = \frac{33.33\,oz}{1\,qt} \quad x = 49.995\,oz$$

40. 75 mg = __1.25__ gr

$$\frac{X\,gr}{75\,mg} = \frac{1\,gr}{60\,mg} \quad 60x = 75 \quad x = 1.25\,gr$$

41. 18 gr = __1080__ mg

$$\frac{X\,mg}{18\,gr} = \frac{60\,mg}{1\,gr} \quad x = 1080$$

42. 0.25 qt = __250__ ml

$$\frac{X\,mL}{0.25\,qt} = \frac{1000\,mL}{1\,qt} \quad x = 250\,mL$$

43. 1.05 pt = __33.6__ T

$$\frac{X\,T}{480\,mL} = \frac{1\,T}{15\,mL} \quad 15x = 480 \quad x = 32\,T \quad \boxed{so\ 1\,pt = 32\,T}$$

$$\frac{X\,T}{1.05\,pt} = \frac{32\,T}{1\,pt} \quad x = 33.6\,T$$

44. 540 oz = __16.2__ qt

$$\frac{X\,qt}{540\,oz} = \frac{1\,qt}{33.33\,oz} \quad 33.33x = 540 \quad x = 16.2\,qt$$

45. 3.6 pt = __345.6__ t

$$\frac{X\,t}{3.6\,pt} = \frac{96\,t}{1\,pt} \quad x = 345.6\,t$$

Rx Success™ Complete Guide to Medical Math

Chapter Nine

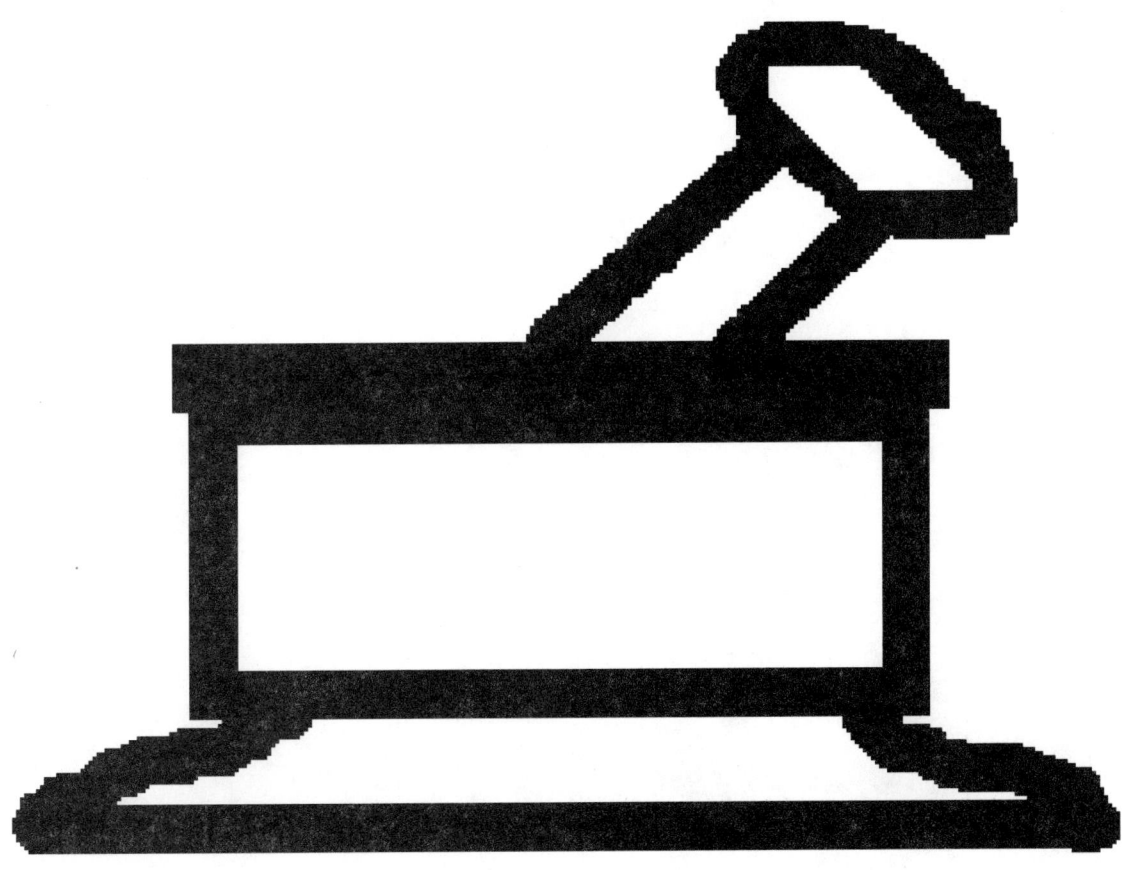

Dosage Calculations

Rx Success™ Complete Guide to Medical Math

Dosage Calculations – Step One

Calculating doses for patients can involve several steps, depending on how the medication is ordered. Each step is presented individually in the pages that follow. Finally, at the end of the section, homework problems will be presented that require all of the steps to solve. Read the problems carefully! Certain steps may need to be performed in a different order than presented.

Step One – Calculating Volume.
When a medication is ordered for a patient, it is not enough to simply know how much drug the patient needs. Often the medication is in a liquid dosage form, whether it is oral or injectable. This means that you must calculate how many mls of liquid to give the patient. To perform this calculation, you must know the *concentration* of the drug. This value represents how much drug is in a specific volume of the liquid. The concentration will usually be given as a fraction (i.e. 20 mg/ml).

$$\frac{20 \text{ mg}}{1 \text{ ml}} \quad \text{is equal to…} \quad \textbf{20 mg of drug per 1 ml of liquid}$$

If this value is *not* given as a fraction, it must be converted to a fraction before performing the calculation.

Suppose a patient needs 75 mg of a drug. This particular drug is only available as a liquid. Since you cannot "pour out" 75 mg of a drug, you must use the concentration of the drug as the code, for the calculation. This calculation will determine how many mls of liquid will deliver exactly 75 mg of drug.

Use the following Sample Problems as a guide to complete the Tutor Sheets™ and homework problems that follow.

Rx Success™ Complete Guide to Medical Math

Dosage Calculations - Step One Sample Problems

1. **Order:** metoprolol 5 mg sq every morning

   Supply: metoprolol 100 mg per 1 ml

   How many ml does the patient need per day?

   Handwritten: $\frac{X\,mL}{5\,mg} = \frac{1\,mL}{100\,mg}$ $100X = 5$ $X = 0.05\,mL$

   Solution: $\frac{5\,mg}{X\,ml} = \frac{100\,mg}{1\,ml}$

   Now cross multiply to get: $100X = 5$ then divide both sides by 100 to isolate X and we get

   $X = \frac{5}{100}$

   Convert 5/100 to a decimal by dividing down and the final answer is

   X = 0.05 ml

---

2. **Order:** A patient is to receive 400 mg Cefzil® suspension, by mouth two times daily for ten days. The suspension is available as 250 mg/5 ml.

   How many mls are needed for *one dose*?

   Solution: $\frac{250\,mg}{5\,ml} = \frac{400\,mg}{X\,ml}$

   Handwritten: $\frac{X\,mL}{400\,mg} = \frac{5\,mL}{250\,mg}$ $250X = 2000$ $X = 8\,mL$

   Now, cross multiply to get **X = 8 ml**

   Handwritten: $\frac{X\,mL}{400\,mg} = \frac{5\,mL}{250\,mg}$ $250X = 2000$ $X = 8\,mL$

Rx Success™ Complete Guide to Medical Math

3. Order: The patient needs 60 mEq of potassium chloride (KCl). KCl is available as 20 mEq/ml.

   How many total mls of KCl are needed?

   Solution: $\dfrac{20\text{ mEq}}{1\text{ ml}} = \dfrac{60\text{ mEq}}{X\text{ ml}}$

   Now, cross multiply to get X = 3 ml

---

4. Order: 30 mg of ketorolac has been ordered every six hours, for 24 hours. Ketorolac is available as 15mg/ml.

   How many total mls of ketorolac are needed in the 24 hour period?

   Solution: $\dfrac{15\text{ mg}}{1\text{ ml}} = \dfrac{30\text{ mg}}{X\text{ ml}}$

   Now, cross multiply to get X = 2 ml. This tells us that the patient needs two ml of ketorolac per dose. We know that the patient receives a dose every six hours. In a 24 hour period the patient will receive four doses of medication. The final step is to multiply the total number of doses the patient receives in a 24 hours period by the total number of ml per dose.

   $$\underset{\text{total \# of doses}}{4} \times \underset{\text{mls per dose}}{2} = \underset{\text{total \# of mls}}{8}$$

Page - 114

Rx Success™ Complete Guide to Medical Math
Dosage Calculations - Step One Tutor Sheets™

USE THIS WORKSHEET AS A GUIDE TO HELP YOU SOLVE THE HOMEWORK PROBLEMS!

1. A patient is to receive 350 mg of a drug per dose. The drug is available as 500 mg/2.5 ml. How many mls are needed for each dose?

    Solution: $\dfrac{500 \text{ mg}}{2.5 \text{ ml}} = \dfrac{350 \text{ mg}}{X \text{ ml}}$ (cross-multiply)

    $\dfrac{X \text{ mL}}{350 \text{ mg}} = \dfrac{2.5 \text{ mL}}{500 \text{ mg}}$

    $500 x = 875$

    $x = 1.75 \text{ mL}$

    _____ = _____

    Answer: X = _____ ml

2. The strength of a drug is 3.75 mg/ml. A patient is ordered to receive 15 mg of the drug per dose. How many mls does the patient need for one dose?

    Solution: $\dfrac{3.75 \text{ mg}}{1 \text{ ml}} = \dfrac{15 \text{ mg}}{X \text{ ml}}$ (cross-multiply)

    $\dfrac{X \text{ mL}}{15 \text{ mg}} = \dfrac{1 \text{ mL}}{3.75 \text{ mg}}$

    $3.75 x = 15$

    $x = 4 \text{ mL}$

    _____ = _____

    Answer: X = _____ ml

3. The strength of a drug is 50 mcg/ml. A patient is ordered to receive 175 mcg of the drug per dose. How many mls does the patient need for one dose?

    Solution: $\dfrac{50 \text{ mcg}}{1 \text{ ml}} = \dfrac{175 \text{ mg}}{X \text{ ml}}$ (cross-multiply)

    $\dfrac{X \text{ mL}}{175 \text{ mcg}} = \dfrac{1 \text{ mL}}{50 \text{ mcg}}$

    $50 x = 175$

    $x = 3.5 \text{ mL}$

    _____ = _____

    Answer: X = _____ ml

Rx Success™ Complete Guide to Medical Math

4. Heparin solution is available in a strength of 40,000 units/ml. A patient is to receive 25,000 units of heparin in 500 ml of 5% Dextrose in Water. How many mls of heparin solution are needed?

   Solution: _____ = _____

   $$\frac{X\ mL}{25000} = \frac{1\ mL}{40000}$$

   _____ = _____

   $$40000 X = 25000$$
   $$X = 0.625\ mL$$

   Answer: X = _____ ml

5. Naloxone is available as 0.4 mg/ml. A patient is to receive a 300 mcg dose. How many mls of naloxone solution are needed?

   Solution: First, either convert 0.4 mg into mcg *or* convert 300 mcg into mg. This ensures that your cross multiplication problem is set up properly with units matching across the top and bottom.

   $$\frac{X\ mL}{0.3\ mg} = \frac{1\ mL}{0.4\ mg}$$

   $$0.4 X = 0.3$$
   $$X = 0.75\ mL$$

   | ____mg / 1 ml = ____mg / X ml | **OR** | ____mcg / 1 ml = ____mcg / X ml |

   _____ = _____   _____ = _____

   Answer: X = _____ ml

6. A drug is available as 1.25 g per 10 ml. A patient is to receive a 75 mg dose twice daily for three days. How many mls of solution are needed to fill the entire order?

   Solution: First, either convert 1.25 g into mg *or* convert 75 mg into g. This ensures that your cross multiplication problem is set up properly with units matching across the top and bottom.

   | ____g / 10 ml = ____g / X ml | **OR** | ____mg / 10 ml = ____mg / X ml |

Rx Success™ Complete Guide to Medical Math

_____ = _____   _____ = _____

Answer: X = _____ml

Finally, you must calculate how much is needed for the entire order. The problem states that the patient is to receive a dose twice daily for 3 days. Calculate how many total doses are given to the patient.

$$\underset{\text{\# of doses per day}}{_____} \times \underset{\text{total \# of days}}{_____} = \underset{\text{total \# of doses}}{_____}$$

Now, multiply the total number of doses by the number of mls needed for each dose. This will give the total number of mls needed to fill the entire order.

$$\underset{\text{total \# of doses}}{_____} \times \underset{\text{mls per dose}}{_____} = \underset{\text{total \# of mls}}{_____}$$

$$\frac{X \, mL}{450 \, mg} = \frac{10 \, mL}{1250 \, mg}$$

$$1250 \, x = 4500$$

$$x = 3.6 \, mL$$

Answers to Tutor Sheets™ Calculations
1) 1.75 ml   2) 4 ml   3) 3.5 ml   4) 0.625 ml   5) 0.75 ml   6) 3.6 ml

Rx Success™ Complete Guide to Medical Math

Dosage Calculations Step One - Homework

Using fractions and cross multiplication, calculate the following doses. Round answers to the nearest hundredth.

1. Penicillin suspension is available as 250 mg/5 ml. A patient is ordered to receive 375 mg three times daily. How many mls are needed for one dose?

$$\frac{X\,mL}{375\,mg} = \frac{5\,mL}{250\,mg} \qquad \frac{X\,mL}{375\,mg} = \frac{5\,mL}{250\,mg} \qquad 250x = 1875$$
$$250x = 1875 \qquad\qquad x = 7.5\,mL$$
$$x = 7.5\,mL$$

___7.5___ ml

2. The ordered dosage of a drug is 15 mg. The drug is available as 30 mg per 2 ml. How many mls are needed?

$$\frac{X\,mL}{15\,mg} = \frac{2\,mL}{30\,mg} \qquad \frac{15\,mg}{X\,ml} = \frac{30\,mg}{2\,ml}$$
$$30x = 30 \qquad\qquad 30 = 30x$$
$$x = 1\,mL \qquad\qquad x = 1$$

___1___ ml

3. The drug is available as 0.4 mg/ml. The physician has ordered a dose of 0.3 mg for a patient weighing 86 kg. How many mls of solution are needed?

$$\frac{X\,mL}{0.3\,mg} = \frac{1\,mL}{0.4\,mg} \qquad \frac{0.4\,mg}{1\,ml} = \frac{0.3\,mg}{X\,ml}$$
$$0.4x = 0.3 \qquad\qquad 0.4x = 0.3$$
$$x = 0.75\,mL \qquad\qquad x = 0.75\,ml$$

___0.75___ ml

4. The drug is available as 1000 U per 1.5 ml. A 1500 U dose is ordered.

$$\frac{X\,mL}{1500\,U} = \frac{1.5\,mL}{1000\,U} \qquad \frac{X\,mL}{1500\,U} = \frac{1.5\,mL}{1000\,U} \qquad 1000x = 2250$$
$$1000x = 2250 \qquad\qquad x = 2.25\,mL$$
$$x = 2.25\,mL$$

___2.25___ ml

5. The concentration of potassium chloride (KCl) solution is 20 mEq per ml. The patient needs 75 mEq of potassium chloride in 1000 ml of D5W. How many mls of KCl solution are needed to prepare this order?

$$\frac{X\,mL}{75\,mEq} = \frac{1\,mL}{20\,mEq} \qquad \frac{20\,mEq}{1\,mL} = \frac{75\,mEq\;in\;1000\,mL\,of\,D5W}{X\,mL}$$
$$20x = 75 \qquad\qquad 20x = 75$$
$$x = 3.75\,mL \qquad\qquad x = 3.75\,mL$$

___3.75___ ml

6. Prepare a 70 mg dose from a solution labeled 100 mg/2 ml.

$$\frac{X\,mL}{70\,mg} = \frac{2\,mL}{100\,mg} \qquad \frac{100\,mg}{2\,mL} = \frac{70\,mg}{X\,ml}$$
$$100x = 140 \qquad\qquad 100x = 140$$
$$x = 1.4\,mL \qquad\qquad x = 1.4$$

___1.4___ ml

Rx Success™ Complete Guide to Medical Math

7. Potassium chloride is available 20 mEq per 2 ml. Prepare a dose of 7.5 mEq.

$\frac{X\,mL}{7.5\,mEq} = \frac{2\,mL}{20\,mEq}$

$20x = 15$
$x = 0.75\,mL$

$\frac{X\,mL}{7.5\,mEq} = \frac{2\,mL}{20\,mEq}$ $20x = 15$ $x = 0.75\,mL$

__0.75__ ml

8. An IV solution is labeled 20 mEq/10 ml. Draw up an 80 mEq dose from this solution.

$\frac{X\,mL}{80\,mEq} = \frac{10\,mL}{20\,mEq}$
$20x = 800$
$x = 40\,mL$

$\frac{X\,mL}{80\,mEq} = \frac{10\,mL}{20\,mEq}$ $20x = 800$ $x = 40$

__40__ ml

9. A 2.5 mg dose of a drug has been ordered for a 110 lb patient. The drug is labeled 0.01 g/ml. How many mls are needed?

$\frac{X\,mL}{2.5\,mg} = \frac{1\,mL}{10\,mg}$
$10x = 2.5$
$x = 0.25\,mL$

$\frac{X\,mL}{2.5\,mg} = \frac{1\,mL}{10\,mg}$ $10x = 2.5$ $x = 0.25\,mL$

__0.25__ ml

10. A patient is to receive 200 mEq of sodium bicarbonate from a solution labeled 50 mEq per 50 ml. How many mls of solution are needed?

$\frac{X\,mL}{200\,mEq} = \frac{50\,mL}{50\,mEq}$
$50x = 10000$
$x = 200\,mL$

$\frac{X\,mL}{200\,mEq} = \frac{50\,mL}{50\,mEq}$ $50x = 10000$ $x = 200$

__200__ ml

11. A solution is labeled 40 mg/ml. How many mg of drug are in 20 mls of this solution?

$\frac{X\,mg}{20\,mL} = \frac{40\,mg}{1\,mL}$
$x = 800\,mg$

$\frac{X\,mg}{20\,mL} = \frac{40\,mg}{1\,mL}$ $x = 800\,mg$

__800__ mg

12. Naloxone is available as 400 mcg per ml. If a patient receives 0.8 ml, how many mg of drug have they been given?

$\frac{X\,mg}{0.8\,mL} = \frac{0.4\,mg}{1\,mL}$
$x = 0.32\,mg$

$\frac{X\,mg}{0.8\,mL} = \frac{0.4\,mg}{1\,mL}$ $x = 0.32\,mg$

__0.32__ mg

13. A drug is labeled 50 mg/10 ml. How many mls are required to provide an 8 mg dose?

$\frac{X\,mL}{8\,mg} = \frac{10\,mL}{50\,mg}$
$50x = 80$
$x = 1.6\,mL$

$\frac{X\,mL}{8\,mg} = \frac{10\,mL}{50\,mg}$ $50x = 80$ $x = 1.6\,mL$

__1.6__ ml

Rx Success™ Complete Guide to Medical Math

14. An IV solution is labeled "KCl 10 mEq/5 ml". The entire bag is 50 ml. How many mEq of KCl are in the entire bag?

$$\frac{x \text{ mEq}}{50 \text{ mL}} = \frac{10 \text{ mEq}}{5 \text{ mL}}$$

$5x = 500$
$x = 100 \text{ mEq}$

___100___ mEq

15. A 10 ml vial is labeled "5 mg/2 ml". How many mg of drug are in the entire vial?

$$\frac{x \text{ mg}}{10 \text{ mL}} = \frac{5 \text{ mg}}{2 \text{ mL}}$$

$2x = 50$
$x = 25 \text{ mg}$

___25___ mg

16. Gentamicin is available as 40 mg per ml. Prepare a dose of 275 mg.

$$\frac{x \text{ mL}}{275 \text{ mg}} = \frac{1 \text{ mL}}{40 \text{ mg}}$$

$40x = 275$
$x = 6.875 \text{ mL}$

___6.875___ ml

17. A drug is available as 120 mg per 2 ml. If a patient receives 1.2 ml, how many mg of drug have they been given?

$$\frac{x \text{ mg}}{1.2 \text{ mL}} = \frac{120 \text{ mg}}{2 \text{ mL}}$$

$2x = 144$
$x = 72 \text{ mg}$

___72___ mg

18. A patient is to receive 400 mg of a drug labeled 0.25 g/5 ml. The patient was given 12 ml. Is this correct? If not, how many mls *should* the patient have received?

$$0.25 \text{ g} \cdot \frac{1000 \text{ mg}}{\text{g}} = \frac{250 \text{ mg}}{5 \text{ mL}} = \frac{400 \text{ mg}}{x \text{ mL}}$$

$250x = 2000$
$x = 8 \text{ mL}$

YES or (NO)   ___8___ ml

$$\frac{x \text{ mL}}{400 \text{ mg}} = \frac{5 \text{ mL}}{250 \text{ mg}}$$
$250x = 2000$
$x = 8 \text{ mL}$

19. A patient is to receive 8 mg of a drug labeled 5 mg/ml. The patient was given 1.6 ml. Is this correct? If not, how many mls *should* the patient have received?

$$\frac{x \text{ mL}}{8 \text{ mg}} = \frac{1 \text{ mL}}{5 \text{ mg}}$$

$5x = 8$
$x = 1.6 \text{ mL}$

(YES) or NO   _____ ml

$$\frac{x \text{ mL}}{8 \text{ mg}} = \frac{1 \text{ mL}}{5 \text{ mg}}$$
$5x = 8$
$x = 1.6 \text{ mL}$

20. Draw up a 9 mg dose from a bottle labeled 15 mg in 5 ml.

$$\frac{15 \text{ mg}}{5 \text{ mL}} = \frac{9 \text{ mg}}{x \text{ mL}}$$

$15x = 45$
$x = 3 \text{ mL}$

___3___ ml

$$\frac{x \text{ mL}}{9 \text{ mg}} = \frac{5 \text{ mL}}{15 \text{ mg}}$$
$15x = 45$
$x = 3 \text{ mL}$

Rx Success™ Complete Guide to Medical Math

21. A patient is to receive 30 mg of a drug. The label says, "25 mg/ml". The patient receives 1.5 ml. Is this correct? If not, how many mls should the patient receive?

$$\frac{X\ mL}{30\ mg} = \frac{1\ mL}{25\ mg} \qquad 25x = 30 \qquad x = 1.2\ mL$$

YES or (NO)   __1.2__ ml

22. A patient is to receive 450,000 U of a drug. The available stock solution is 300,000 U in 1.5 ml. How many mls are required to fill this order?

$$\frac{X\ mL}{450{,}000\ U} = \frac{1.5\ mL}{300{,}000} \qquad 300000x = 675000 \qquad x = 2.25\ mL$$

__2.25__ ml

23. A drug is available as 0.2 g/5 ml. Draw up a 175 mg dose.

$$\frac{X\ mL}{175\ mg} = \frac{5\ mL}{200\ mg} \qquad 200x = 875 \qquad x = 4.375\ mL$$

__4.375__ ml

24. A patient is given 1.75 mls of a 300 mcg/ml solution. How many mg of drug did the patient receive?

$$\frac{X\ mcg}{1.75\ mL} = \frac{300\ mcg}{1\ mL} \qquad x = 525\ mcg / 1000 = 0.525\ mg$$

__0.525__ mg

25. A patient is given 50 mls of a solution labeled 20 mEq/10 ml. How many mEq of drug did the patient receive?

$$\frac{X\ mEq}{50\ mL} = \frac{20\ mEq}{10\ mL} \qquad 10x = 1000 \qquad x = 100\ mEq$$

__100__ mEq

26. Prepare a 150 mg dose from a vial labeled 0.25 g/25 ml.

$$\frac{X\ mL}{150\ mg} = \frac{25\ mL}{250\ mg} \qquad 250x = 3750 \qquad x = 15\ mL$$

__15__ ml

27. A 10 mg dose of a drug has been ordered. Prepare this dose from a bottle labeled 4000 mcg/ml.

$$\frac{X\ mL}{10\ mg} = \frac{1\ mL}{4\ mg} \qquad 4x = 10 \qquad x = 2.5\ mL$$

__2.5__ ml

Rx Success™ Complete Guide to Medical Math

28. A 75 U dose has been ordered for a patient. The patient is given 1.5 mls from a vial labeled 250 U/2 ml. Did the patient receive the correct dose? If not, how many mls of solution *should* they have received?

$$\frac{X\, mL}{75\, U} = \frac{2\, mL}{250\, U} \qquad 250x = 150 \qquad x = 0.6\, mL$$

YES or (NO)   __0.6__ ml

29. A 450 mcg dose has been ordered for a patient. The patient is given 3 mls from a vial labeled 0.2 mg/2 ml. Did the patient receive the correct dose? If not, how many mls of solution *should* they have received?

$$\frac{X\, mL}{450\, mcg} = \frac{2\, mL}{200\, mcg} \qquad 200x = 900 \qquad x = 4.5\, mL$$

YES or (NO)   __4.5__ ml

30. A drug is available as 1.5 g per 10 ml. A patient is to receive a 500 mg dose three times daily for seven days. How many mls of solution are needed to fill the entire order?

$$\frac{X\, mL}{500\, mg} = \frac{10\, mL}{1500\, mg} \qquad 1500x = 5000 \qquad x = 3.33\, mL \qquad \times 21 = 69.93\, mL$$

__69.93__ ml

31. A patient is to receive 500 mg of drug intravenously every 12 hours for 3 days. The IV solution is labeled 100 mg per 50 ml. How many total mls of solution will be used to fill the entire order?

$$\frac{X\, mL}{500\, mg} = \frac{50\, mL}{100\, mg} \qquad 100x = 25000 \qquad x = 250\, mL \qquad \times 6 = 1500\, mL$$

__1500__ ml

32. A patient is to receive 1.5 mg of drug every 6 hours for 14 days. The drug is available as 750 mcg per 2 ml. How many mls of solution are needed to fill the entire order?

$$\frac{X\, mL}{1.5\, mg} = \frac{2\, mL}{0.75\, mg} \qquad 0.75x = 3 \qquad x = 4\, mL \qquad \times 56 = 224\, mL$$

__224__ ml

33. A patient has been administered 3.75 mls of an amoxicillin suspension labeled 250 mg/5 ml, three times daily for 7 days. How many mg of amoxicillin did the patient receive in total?

____3937.5____ mg

34. A patient has received 2.5 mls of a solution labeled 50 mcg/ml, every four hours for six days. How many mg of drug did the patient receive in total?

____4.5____ mg

35. A 250 ml bag of D5W is labeled, "Vancomycin, 4 mg/ml". The patient received 150 mls of this solution. How many mg of vancomycin were administered to the patient?

____600____ mg

Rx Success™ Complete Guide to Medical Math

Dosage Calculations - Step Two

Step Two – Calculating Doses Using Body Weight
Occasionally a physician will base the amount of drug, ordered for patient, on the patient's body weight. This means that a patient who weighs more requires more drug than a patient who weighs less. This is particularly useful for children and critically ill patients who are receiving injectable medication.

For the most part, body weight is still measured in pounds. However, the dosage recommendations for drugs are usually based on a body weight measured in kilograms. For this reason, medical personnel must be able to convert back and forth between pounds (lbs) and kilograms (kg). For example, an order may say that a patient is to receive 5 mg/kg. This means that the patient must get 5 mg of drug for every 1 kg of body weight. In order to calculate the correct dose for this particular patient, the body weight must be in kilograms, *not* pounds.

When calculating dosages based on weight, the calculations will follow a certain order based on the information given in the problem. Reading over the following steps will help to familiarize you with this order. Then, read over the Sample Problems and complete the Tutor Sheets™ and the homework that follows to perfect these skills. Do not forget to memorize the following conversion factor!

Body Weight Conversion Factor

2.2 lbs = 1 kg

Weight Based Dosage Calculations

1. First, convert the patient's weight into kilograms using this conversion factor: 2.2 lbs = 1 kg. If the patient's weight is given to you in kilograms, skip to step 2.

2. Next, use the physician's order as the "code" for a cross multiplication problem, to determine how much drug the patient needs, based on their body weight.

3. This step involves the concentration of the drug itself. Once the amount of drug needed is calculated (generally in mg, mcg or grams) you may be required to obtain the drug from a bottle. To illustrate this, suppose step 2 says that the patient needs 300 mg of drug, based on his/her body weight. However, the drug is a liquid. It would be impossible to "pour out" 300 mg! When a drug is in a liquid form, it must be dealt with in units of liquid measurement, like milliliters or liters. To calculate the amount of solution needed, the concentration of the drug is needed. Usually the concentration will look something like this: 150 mg/2 ml or

0.25 mg/ml. Use the concentration of the drug as the code for a cross multiplication problem to determine the volume of drug needed to fill the order for the patient.

Rx Success™ Complete Guide to Medical Math

Dosage Calculations - Step Two Sample Problems

Examples:

1. 27 lb = _____ kg

   $$\frac{2.2 \text{ lb}}{1 \text{ kg}} \times \frac{27 \text{ lb}}{X \text{ kg}}$$

   $$\frac{2.2X}{2.2} = \frac{27}{2.2}$$

   $$X = \frac{27}{2.2}$$

   X = 12.27 kg

2. 193 lb = _____ kg

   $$\frac{2.2 \text{ lb}}{1 \text{ kg}} \times \frac{193 \text{ lb}}{X \text{ kg}}$$

   $$\frac{2.2X}{2.2} = \frac{193}{2.2}$$

   $$X = \frac{193}{2.2}$$

   X = 87.72 kg

3. 76 kg = _____ lb

   $$\frac{2.2 \text{ lb}}{1 \text{ kg}} \times \frac{X \text{ lb}}{76 \text{ kg}}$$

   X = 167.2 lb

4. 103 kg = _____ lb

Rx Success™ Complete Guide to Medical Math

$$\frac{2.2 \text{ lb}}{1 \text{ kg}} \underset{}{=} \frac{X \text{ lb}}{103 \text{ kg}}$$

X = 226.6 lb

---

5. A patient is to receive 25 mg/kg per dose. The patient weighs 57 kg.

   How many milligrams will the patient receive?

   Since the patient's weight is given to us in kg, we do *not* need to first convert from lb to kg

   $$\frac{25 \text{ mg}}{1 \text{ kg}} = \frac{X \text{ mg}}{57 \text{ kg}}$$

   $\frac{X \text{ mg}}{57 \text{ kg}} = \frac{25 \text{ mg}}{1 \text{ kg}} \quad X = 1425 \text{ mg}$

   $\frac{X \text{ mg}}{57 \text{ kg}} = \frac{25 \text{ mg}}{1 \text{ kg}}$

   $X = 1425 \text{ mg}$

   X = 1425 mg

---

6. A 15 kg patient is to receive 3 mg per kg of a drug.

   How many milligrams will the patient receive?

   Since the patient's weight is given to us in kg, we do *not* need to first convert from lb to kg

   $\frac{X \text{ mg}}{15 \text{ kg}} = \frac{3 \text{ mg}}{1 \text{ kg}}$
   $X = 45 \text{ mg}$

   $$\frac{3 \text{ mg}}{1 \text{ kg}} = \frac{X \text{ mg}}{15 \text{ kg}}$$

   $\frac{X \text{ mg}}{15 \text{ kg}} = \frac{3 \text{ mg}}{1 \text{ kg}} \quad X = 45 \text{ mg}$

   X = 45 mg

---

7. **Order:** 12 mg/kg per dose
   Patient: 110 lb

   $\frac{X \text{ kg}}{110 \text{ lb}} = \frac{1 \text{ kg}}{2.2 \text{ lb}}$
   $2.2 X = 110$
   $X = 50 \text{ kg}$

   $\frac{X \text{ mg}}{50 \text{ kg}} = \frac{12 \text{ mg}}{1 \text{ kg}} \quad X = 600 \text{ mg}$

   How many milligrams will the patient receive?

   This is a two step problem. Since the order requires that the patent's weight is in kilograms, we must first convert 110 lbs into kilograms. Then we can calculate the dose needed.

Rx Success™ Complete Guide to Medical Math

a. $\dfrac{2.2\ \text{lb}}{1\ \text{kg}} \times\!=\!\times \dfrac{110\ \text{lb}}{X\ \text{kg}}$

$\dfrac{\cancel{2.2}\,X}{\cancel{2.2}} = \dfrac{110}{2.2}$

X = 50 kg

We found that the patient's weight is 50 kg. Now, we can find how much drug is needed in milligrams. The order says to give 12 mg per 1 kg.

b. $\dfrac{12\ \text{mg}}{1\ \text{kg}} = \dfrac{X\ \text{mg}}{50\ \text{kg}}$

X = 600 mg

---

8. **Order:** 7 mg/kg per dose
   Patient: 163 lb

   $\dfrac{X\ kg}{163\ lb} = \dfrac{1\ kg}{2.2\ lb}$ $2.2x = 163$ $\dfrac{X\ mg}{74.09\ kg} = \dfrac{7\ mg}{1\ kg}$ $X = 518.63\ mg$
                             $X = 74.09\ kg$

   How many milligrams will the patient receive?

   First, convert pounds (lb) to kilograms (kg).

   a. $\dfrac{2.2\ \text{lb}}{1\ \text{kg}} \times\!=\!\times \dfrac{163\ \text{lb}}{X\ \text{kg}}$

   $\dfrac{\cancel{2.2}\,X}{\cancel{2.2}} = \dfrac{163}{2.2}$

   $\dfrac{X\ kg}{163\ lb} = \dfrac{1\ kg}{2.2\ lb}$

   $2.2x = 163$
   $x = 74.09\ kg$

   $\dfrac{X\ mg}{74.09\ kg} = \dfrac{7\ mg}{1\ kg}$

   $X = 518.63\ mg$

   X = 74.09 kg

   Now find the dose:

   b. $\dfrac{7\ \text{mg}}{1\ \text{kg}} = \dfrac{X\ \text{mg}}{74.09\ \text{kg}}$

   X = 518.63 mg

Rx Success™ Complete Guide to Medical Math

Dosage Calculations - Step Two Tutor Sheets™

USE THIS WORKSHEET AS A GUIDE TO HELP YOU SOLVE THE HOMEWORK PROBLEMS!

1. 45 lb = _____ kg   Code: 2.2 lb = 1 kg

   $\dfrac{X \text{ kg}}{45 \text{ lb}} = \dfrac{1 \text{ kg}}{2.2 \text{ lb}}$

   $2.2x = 45$

   $x = 20.45 \text{ kg}$

   $\dfrac{2.2 \text{ lb}}{1 \text{ kg}} = \underline{\qquad}$

   $\dfrac{X \text{ kg}}{45 \text{ lb}} = \dfrac{1 \text{ kg}}{2.2 \text{ lb}}$

   $2.2x = 45$

   $x = 20.45 \text{ kg}$

   $\dfrac{2.2 \text{ lb}}{1 \text{ kg}} \times \dfrac{45 \text{ lb}}{X \text{ kg}}$

   $\dfrac{2.2 X}{2.2} = \dfrac{45}{2.2}$

   X = _____

---

2. 12 lb = _____ kg   Code: 2.2 lb = 1 kg

   $\dfrac{X \text{ kg}}{12 \text{ lb}} = \dfrac{1 \text{ kg}}{2.2 \text{ lb}}$

   $2.2x = 12$

   $x = 5.45 \text{ kg}$

   $\dfrac{X \text{ kg}}{12 \text{ lb}} = \dfrac{1 \text{ kg}}{2.2 \text{ lb}}$

   $2.2x = 12$

   $x = 5.45 \text{ kg}$

   _____ = _____

   _____ = _____

   X = _____

---

3. 120 kg = _____ lb   Code: _____ = _____

   $\dfrac{X \text{ lb}}{120 \text{ kg}} = \dfrac{2.2 \text{ lb}}{1 \text{ kg}}$

   $x = 264 \text{ lb}$

   $\dfrac{X \text{ lb}}{120 \text{ kg}} = \dfrac{2.2 \text{ lb}}{X \text{ kg}}$

   $x = 264 \text{ lb}$

   _____ = _____

Rx Success™ Complete Guide to Medical Math

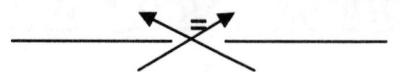

X = _____

---

4. A 78.5 lb patient is to receive 0.3 mg/kg per dose. How many mg are needed for one dose?

Handwritten work:
$\frac{X\ kg}{78.5\ lb} = \frac{1\ kg}{2.2\ lb}$
$2.2x = 78.5$
$x = 35.68\ kg$

$\frac{X\ mg}{35.68\ kg} = \frac{0.3\ mg}{1\ kg}$ $x = 10.704\ mg$

Step One: Convert the patient's weight to kg using the code: 2.2 lb = 1 kg

$\frac{2.2\ lb}{1\ kg} = \frac{78.5\ lb}{X\ kg}$

_____ = _____

X = _____ kg

Handwritten work:
$\frac{X\ kg}{78.5\ lb} = \frac{1\ kg}{2.2\ lb}$
$2.2x = 78.5$
$x = 35.68\ kg$

$\frac{X\ mg}{35.68\ kg} = \frac{0.3}{1\ kg}$
$x = 10.70\ mg$

Step Two: Use the order as the code to determine how many mg the patient needs, based on his/her weight.

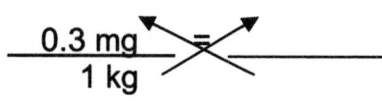
$\frac{0.3\ mg}{1\ kg}$

_____ = _____

X = _____ mg

---

5. A 112 lb patient is to receive 75 mg/kg per day in three equally divided doses. How many mg are needed for one dose?

Handwritten work:
$\frac{X\ kg}{112\ lb} = \frac{1\ kg}{2.2\ lb}$
$2.2x = 112$
$x = 50.91\ kg$

$\frac{X\ mg}{50.91\ kg} = \frac{75\ mg}{1\ kg}$
$x = 3818.25\ mg / 3 = 1272.75\ mg$

Step One: Convert the patient's weight to kg using the code: 2.2 lb = 1 kg

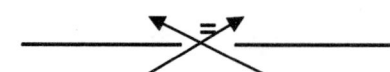

Page - 132

Rx Success™ Complete Guide to Medical Math

_____ = _____

X = _____ kg

Step Two: Use the order (75 mg/kg) as the code to determine how many mg the patient needs, *per day*, based on his/her weight.

$\frac{X \, kg}{112 \, lb} = \frac{1 \, kg}{2.2 \, lb}$

$2.2X = 112$

$X = 50.91 \, kg$

$\frac{X \, mg}{50.91 \, kg} = \frac{25 \, mg}{1 \, kg}$

$X = 1272.75 \, mg$

_____ = _____

X = _____ mg per day

Step Three: Remember, the order said that the amount of drug per day needs to be divided into *three, equal doses*. This requires us to divide the total number of mg (per day) by three. This will tell us how many mg are in just one dose.

_____ divided by 3 = _____
mg per day   mg per dose

---

6. A 78 lb patient is to receive 150 mcg per kg per dose. The patient is to receive a dose every six hours. The drug is available as 50 mg/ml. How many ml are required for one entire day of treatment?

$\frac{X \, kg}{78 \, lb} = \frac{1 \, kg}{2.2 \, lb}$

$2.2X = 78$

$X = 35.45 \, kg$

Step One: Convert the patient's weight to kg.

$\frac{X \, kg}{78 \, lb} = \frac{1 \, kg}{2.2 \, lb}$

$2.2X = 78$

$X = 35.45 \, kg$

$\frac{X \, mg}{35.45 \, kg} = \frac{0.15 \, mg}{1 \, kg}$

$X = 5.32 \, mg$

_____ = _____

$\frac{X \, mg}{35.45 \, kg} = \frac{0.6 \, mg}{1 \, kg}$ $X = 21.27 \, mg$

$\frac{X \, mL}{21.27 \, mg} = \frac{1 \, mL}{50 \, mg}$

$50X = 21.27$

$X = 0.43 \, mL$

$\frac{X \, mL}{5.32 \, mg} = \frac{1 \, mL}{50 \, mg}$

$50X = 5.32$

$X = 0.11 \, mL \times 4 = 0.43 \, mL$

Page - 133

Rx Success™ Complete Guide to Medical Math

X = _____ kg

Step Two: Use the order as the code to determine how many mcg the patient needs, *per dose*, based on his/her weight.

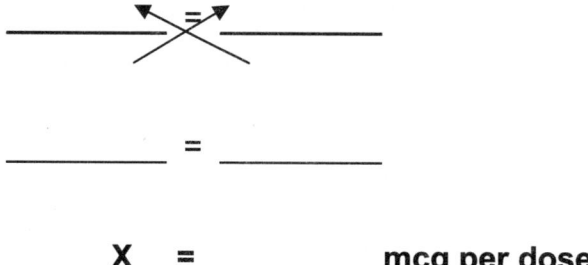

_____ = _____

X = _____ mcg per dose

Step Three: We must calculate how many mls are needed to deliver each dose of medication. Since the amount of drug we found in step is in units of mcg and the concentration of the actual drug in mg, we must first make sure that the two values are in the same units. Either convert the number of **mcg** (found in step 2) into mg *or* convert the concentration (50 **mg**/1 ml) into mcg. This ensures that your cross multiplication problem is set up properly with units matching across the top and bottom.

$$\frac{_____ \text{ mg}}{1 \text{ ml}} = \frac{_____ \text{ mg}}{X \text{ ml}} \quad \text{OR} \quad \frac{_____ \text{ mcg}}{1 \text{ ml}} = \frac{_____ \text{ mcg}}{X \text{ ml}}$$

_____ = _____   _____ = _____

Answer: X = _____ ml per dose

Step Four: The problem asked us to calculate the number of mls needed for an entire day of treatment. Since the patient receives a dose every six hours, he/she will need a total of **four** doses in a 24-hour period of time. This requires us to multiply the total number of ml per dose by four. This will tell us how many ml are needed for one entire day.

_____ multiplied by **4** = _____
ml per dose   ml per day

Rx Success™ Complete Guide to Medical Math

7. A 102 lb patient is to receive 0.1 mg per kg per dose. The patient is to receive a dose every four hours. The drug is available as 500 mcg/ml. How many ml are required for one entire day of treatment?

Step One: Convert the patient's weight to kg.

Handwritten work (left margin):
$$\frac{X\,kg}{102\,lb} = \frac{1\,kg}{2.2\,lb}$$
$$2.2x = 102$$
$$x = 46.36\,kg$$

$$\frac{X\,mg}{46.36\,kg} = \frac{0.1\,mg}{1\,kg}$$
$$x = 4.64\,mg/dose$$

$$\frac{X\,mL}{4640\,mcg} = \frac{1\,mL}{500\,mcg}$$
$$500x = 4640$$
$$x = 9.28\,mL \times 6 = 55.68\,mL$$

_____ ⤫ _____

_____ = _____

X = _____ kg

Step Two: Use the order as the code to determine how many mg the patient needs, *per dose*, based on his/her weight.

_____ ⤫ _____

_____ = _____

X = _____ mg per dose

Handwritten work (right side):
$$\frac{X\,kg}{102\,lb} = \frac{1\,kg}{2.2\,lb}$$
$$2.2x = 102$$
$$x = 46.36\,kg$$

$$\frac{X\,mg}{46.36\,kg} = \frac{0.6\,mg}{1\,kg}$$
$$x = 27.82\,mg$$

$$\frac{X\,mL}{27.82\,mg} = \frac{1\,mL}{0.5\,mg}$$
$$0.5x = 27.82$$
$$x = 55.64\,mL$$

Step Three: Calculate how many ml are needed to deliver each dose of medication. Since the amount of drug we found in step is in units of mg and the concentration of the actual drug in mcg, we must first make sure that the two values are in the same units. Either convert the number of **mg** (found in step 2) into mcg *or* convert the concentration (500 **mcg**/1 ml) into mg. This ensures that your cross multiplication problem is set up properly with units matching across the top and bottom.

$$\frac{\_\_\_\_\,mg}{1\,ml} = \frac{\_\_\_\_\,mg}{X\,ml} \quad\quad OR \quad\quad \frac{\_\_\_\_\,mcg}{1\,ml} = \frac{\_\_\_\_\,mcg}{X\,ml}$$

_____ = _____   _____ = _____

Answer: X = _____ ml per dose

Rx Success™ Complete Guide to Medical Math

Step Four: The problem asked us to calculate the number of mls needed for an entire day of treatment. Since the patient receives a dose every four hours, he/she will need a total of **six** doses in a 24-hour period of time. This requires us to multiply the total number of ml per dose by six. This will tell us how many ml are needed for one entire day.

_____ multiplied by **6** = _____
ml per dose   ml per day

---

8. A 36.2 lb patient is to receive 3 mg/kg of a drug, per day. The patient is to receive this amount in two, equally divided doses for a total of 5 days. The drug is available as 45 mg/3 ml. How many ml are required for one dose?

Step One: Convert the patient's weight to kg.

Handwritten work (left margin):
$$\frac{x \text{ kg}}{36.2 \text{ lb}} = \frac{1 \text{ kg}}{2.2 \text{ lb}}$$
$$2.2x = 36.2$$
$$x = 16.45 \text{ kg}$$

$$\frac{x \text{ mg}}{16.45 \text{ kg}} = \frac{3 \text{ mg}}{1 \text{ kg}}$$
$$x = 49.35 \text{ mg/day}$$

$$\frac{x \text{ mL}}{49.35 \text{ mg}} = \frac{3 \text{ mL}}{45 \text{ mg}}$$
$$45x = 148.05$$
$$x = 3.29 \text{ mL/day} / 2 = 1.65 \text{ mL}$$

_____ ⨯ _____

_____ = _____

X = _____ kg

Step Two: Use the order (3 mg/kg) as the code to determine how many mg the patient needs, **per day**, based on his/her weight.

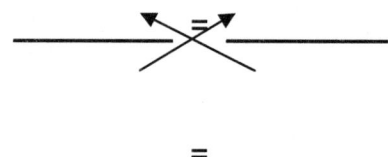

X = _____ mg per day

Step Three: Convert the number of mg (per day) into ml (per day), using the strength of the drug (45 mg/3 ml).

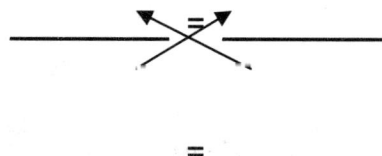

Page - 136

Rx Success™ Complete Guide to Medical Math

X = _____ml per day

Step Four: Since the order states that the patient is to receive the daily dose of medication in *two equally divided doses*, we must divide the number of ml per day into two equal doses. This will determine how many ml the patient will receive *per dose*

_____ divided by **2** = _____
ml per day   ml per dose

Answers to Tutor Sheets™ Calculations
1) 20.45 kg   2) 5.45 kg   3) 264 lb   4) 10.7 mg   5) 1272.75 mg   6) 0.43 ml   7) 55.68 ml   8) 1.65 ml

Rx Success™ Complete Guide to Medical Math

Dosage Calculations - Step Two Homework

Calculate the following body weight equivalents: (round to nearest tenth)

1. Pounds to Kilograms

	Pounds	Kilograms
a)	48 lb	21.82 kg
b)	112 lb	50.91 kg
c)	14 lb	6.36 kg
d)	35.5 lb	16.14 kg
e)	220 lb	100 kg
f)	10.5 lb	4.77 kg
g)	100 lb	45.45 kg
h)	50.1 lb	22.77 kg
i)	23 lb	10.45 kg
j)	103 lb	46.82 kg
k)	2.2 lb	1 kg
l)	30 lb	13.64 kg
m)	18 lb	8.18 kg
n)	178 lb	80.91 kg
o)	168.5 lb	76.59 kg

2. Kilograms to Pounds

	Pounds	Kilograms
a)	220 lbs	100
b)	34.1 lb	15.5
c)	19.8 lb	9
d)	154 lb	70

Rx Success™ Complete Guide to Medical Math

	Pounds	Kilograms
e)	264 lb	120
f)	118.8 lb	54
g)	51.7 lb	23.5
h)	176 lb	80
i)	99 lb	45
j)	57.64 lb	26.2
k)	68.2 lb	31
l)	209 lb	95
m)	169.4 lb	77
n)	180.4 lb	82
o)	83.6 lb	38

Calculate the doses for the patients in the following problems.

3. A 56 kg patient is to receive 1.5 mg/kg of a drug. How many mg are needed?

$$\frac{X\ mg}{56\ kg} = \frac{1.5\ mg}{1\ kg} \quad X = 84\ mg$$

$$\frac{X\ mg}{56\ kg} = \frac{1.5\ mg}{1\ kg}$$
$$X = 84\ mg$$

_____84_____ mg

4. A 15 kg patient is to receive 75 mg/kg of a drug. How many mg are needed?

$$\frac{X\ mg}{15\ kg} = \frac{75\ mg}{1\ kg}$$
$$X = 1125\ mg$$

_____1125_____ mg

5. A 17 kg patient is to receive 22 mg/kg of a drug. How many mg are needed?

$$\frac{X\ mg}{17\ kg} = \frac{22\ mg}{1\ kg}$$
$$X = 374\ mg$$

_____374_____ mg

Rx Success™ Complete Guide to Medical Math

6. An 8.4 kg infant is to receive 0.25 mg/kg of a drug. How many mg are needed?

　　　　　　　　　　　　　　　　　　　　　　　　　　　　　　2.1 mg

7. A 12 year old patient who weighs 40 kg is to receive 0.45 mg/kg of a drug. How many mg are needed?

　　　　　　　　　　　　　　　　　　　　　　　　　　　　　　18 mg

8. A physician has ordered a 127 lb patient to receive 25 mg/kg of a drug, per dose. How many mg are needed for one dose?

$$\frac{x \, mg}{57.73 \, kg} = \frac{25 \, mg}{1 \, kg}$$

$$x = 1443.25$$

　　　　　　　　　　　　　　　　　　　　　　　　　　　　1443.25 mg per dose

9. A 45 lb patient needs 0.02 mg/kg of a drug per dose. How many mg are needed for one dose?

$$\frac{x \, mg}{20.45} = \frac{0.02 \, mg}{1 \, kg}$$

$$x = 0.41 \, mg$$

　　　　　　　　　　　　　　　　　　　　　　　　　　　　0.41 mg per dose

10. A physician has ordered that a 78 lb patient is to receive 20 mg per kg per dose. How many mg are needed for one dose?

$$\frac{x \, kg}{78 \, lb} = \frac{1 \, kg}{2.2 \, lb} \qquad \frac{x \, mg}{35.45 \, kg} = \frac{20 \, mg}{1 \, kg}$$

$$2.2x = 78 \qquad\qquad x = 709 \, mg$$

$$x = 35.45 \, kg$$

　　　　　　　　　　　　　　　　　　　　　　　　　　　　709 mg per dose

11. A 60 lb patient is to receive 0.5 mg/kg per dose of a drug. How many mg are needed for one dose?

$$\frac{x \, mg}{27.27 \, kg} = \frac{0.5 \, mg}{1 \, kg}$$

$$x = 13.64 \, mg$$

　　　　　　　　　　　　　　　　　　　　　　　　　　　　13.64 mg per dose

Rx Success™ Complete Guide to Medical Math

12. A physician orders a patient to receive 10 mg/kg per dose of a drug. The drug is to be administered three times daily. The patient weighs 90 lbs. Calculate how many mg are needed for **one day**.

$\frac{90}{2.2} = 40.91 \text{ kg}$ $\frac{x \text{ mg}}{40.91 \text{ kg}} = \frac{10 \text{ mg}}{1 \text{ kg}}$

$x = 409.1 \text{ mg/dose} \times 3 = 1227.3 \text{ mg/day}$

_1227.3_ mg per day

13. A physician orders a patient to receive 0.25 mg per kg per dose of a drug. The drug is to be administered every 12 hours. The patient weighs 90 lbs. Calculate how many mg are needed for one day.

$\frac{90}{2.2} = 40.91 \text{ kg}$ $\frac{x \text{ mg}}{40.91 \text{ kg}} = \frac{0.25 \text{ mg}}{1 \text{ kg}}$

$x = 10.23 \text{ mg} \times 2 = 20.46 \text{ mg}$

_20.46_ mg per day

14. A 38 lb patient is ordered to receive 1.5 mg/kg of a drug per dose. The patient is administered a dose every 4 hours. How many mg are needed to provide enough drug for two days of treatment?

$\frac{38}{2.2} = 17.27 \text{ kg}$ $\frac{x \text{ mg}}{17.27 \text{ kg}} = \frac{1.5 \text{ mg}}{1 \text{ kg}}$

$x = 25.91 \text{ mg} \times 12 = 310.92 \text{ mg}$

_310.92_ mg for two days

15. A physician has ordered 7.5 mg/kg per day in three equally divided doses. The patient weighs 104 lbs. How many mg of drug are needed for **each dose**?

$\frac{104}{2.2} = 47.27 \text{ kg}$ $\frac{x \text{ mg}}{47.27 \text{ kg}} = \frac{7.5 \text{ mg}}{1 \text{ kg}}$

$x = 354.53 \text{ mg} / 3 = 118.18 \text{ mg}$

_118.18_ mg per dose

16. A 60 lb patient is to receive 0.375 mg per kg per day of a drug. The duration of therapy is 14 days. How many total mg of drug are needed to fill this order?

$\frac{60}{2.2} = 27.27 \text{ kg}$ $\frac{x \text{ mg}}{27.27 \text{ kg}} = \frac{0.375 \text{ mg}}{1 \text{ kg}}$

$x = 10.23 \text{ mg} \times 14 = 143.17 \text{ mg}$

_143.17_ mg

Rx Success™ Complete Guide to Medical Math

17. A physician has ordered a 45 lb child to receive 25 mg per kg per day of a drug, for a total of 10 days. How many total mg of drug are needed to fill this order?

$\frac{45}{2.2} = 20.45 kg$ $\frac{x\,mg}{20.45kg} = \frac{25\,mg}{1\,kg}$

$x = 511.25\,mg \times 10 = 5112.50\,mg$

_____5112.50__ mg

18. A 186 lb patient is to receive 1.25 mg/kg per day of a drug. The drug is to be administered for a total of five days. How many total mg of drug are needed to fill this order?

$\frac{186\,lb}{2.2\,lb} = 84.55\,kg$ $\frac{x\,mg}{84.5\,kg} = \frac{1.25\,mg}{1\,kg}$ $x = 105.63\,mg/day$

$\times\ 5$

528.13

_____528.1__ mg

19. A patient, weighing 85 lbs is ordered to receive 50 mg of a drug every 12 hours for 3 days. How many mg of drug are needed to fill the entire order?

$50 \times 2 \times 3 = 300\,mg\ total$

_____300__ mg

20. A 160 lb patient is to receive 240 mg of a drug every 4 hours for 10 days. How many mg are needed to fill the entire order?

$\frac{24}{4} = 6 \times 10 = 60 \times 240\,mg = 14400$

_____14400__ mg

21. A physician has ordered a 23 kg patient to receive 70 mg/kg of a drug per day in three, equally divided doses. How many mg are needed for one day?

$\frac{x\,mg}{23\,kg} = \frac{70\,mg}{1\,kg}$

$x = 1610\,mg/day$

_____1610__ mg per day

22. You receive an order for a 130 lb patient to receive 500 mg of drug per day in four, equally divided doses. How many mg are needed for each dose?

$500/4 = 125\,mg$

_____125__ mg per dose

Rx Success™ Complete Guide to Medical Math

23. A 58 lb patient is to receive 3.5 mg/kg of a drug in 500 mls of D5W, three times daily. How many mg of drug are needed for each dose?

$\frac{58}{2.2} = 26.36 \text{ kg}$ $\frac{X \text{ mg}}{26.36 \text{ kg}} = \frac{3.5 \text{ mg}}{1 \text{ kg}}$

$X = 92.26 \text{ mg}$

__92.26__ mg per dose

24. The order states that a patient is to receive 150 mcg/kg of a drug. The patient weighs 12 lbs. How many **mg** of drug are needed?

$\frac{12}{2.2} = 5.45 \text{ kg}$ $\frac{X \text{ mcg}}{5.45 \text{ kg}} = \frac{150 \text{ mg}}{1 \text{ kg}}$

$X = 817.5 \text{ mcg} / 1000 = 0.8175 \text{ mg}$

__0.8175__ mg

25. The order reads: 0.25 mg/kg/day in two equally divided doses. The patient weighs 92 lb. How many mg of drug are needed for three days of therapy?

$\frac{92}{2.2} = 41.82 \text{ kg}$ $\frac{X \text{ mg}}{41.82 \text{ kg}} = \frac{0.25 \text{ mg}}{1 \text{ kg}}$

$X = 10.46 \text{ mg/day} \times 3 = 31.37 \text{ mg}$

__31.37__ mg

26. A patient is to receive 50 mcg of drug per kg of body weight, per day. The patient weighs 17 lbs. How many mg are needed for one day?

$\frac{17}{2.2} = 7.73 \text{ kg}$ $\frac{X \text{ mcg}}{7.73 \text{ kg}} = \frac{50 \text{ mcg}}{1 \text{ kg}}$

$X = 386.5 \text{ mcg} / 1000 = 0.3865 \text{ mg}$

__0.3865__ mg per day

27. A patient is to receive 0.05 g per kg per day of a drug, in two equally divided doses. The patient weighs 55 lb. How many mg of drug are needed for each dose?

$\frac{55}{2.2} = 25 \text{ kg}$ $\frac{X \text{ mg}}{25 \text{ kg}} = \frac{50 \text{ mg}}{1 \text{ kg}}$

$X = 1250 \text{ mg}/2 = 625 \text{ mg/dose}$

__625__ mg per dose

28. A 28.5 lb child is to receive 25 mcg of drug per kg every 6 hours. How many mg of drug are needed to fill the order for five days?

$\frac{28.5}{2.2} = 12.95 \text{ kg}$ $\frac{X \text{ mg}}{12.95 \text{ kg}} = \frac{0.025 \text{ mg}}{1 \text{ kg}}$

$X = 0.3238 \text{ mg} \times 4 = 1.295 \text{ mg/day} \times 5 = 6.476 \text{ mg}$

__6.48__ mg

Rx Success™ Complete Guide to Medical Math

29. The order states that a 220 lb patient is to receive 0.75 g/kg/day in two equally divided doses. How many mg are needed per dose?

$\frac{220}{2.2} = 100 \text{ kg}$ $\frac{x \text{ mg}}{100 \text{ kg}} = \frac{750 \text{ mg}}{1 \text{ kg}}$

$x = 75000 \text{ mg/day} \div 2 = 37500 \text{ mg/dose}$

__37500__ mg per dose

30. A 132 lb patient has been given 120 mg of a drug. The dosage range for the drug is between 1.5 mg/kg and 3.8 mg/kg. Is the amount of drug the patient was given within the acceptable limits?

$\frac{132}{2.2} = 60 \text{ kg}$

$\frac{x \text{ mg}}{60 \text{ kg}} = \frac{1.5 \text{ mg}}{1 \text{ kg}}$ $x = 90 \text{ mg}$

$\frac{x \text{ mg}}{60 \text{ kg}} = \frac{3.8 \text{ mg}}{1 \text{ kg}}$ $x = 228 \text{ mg}$

(YES) or NO

31. A 75 lb patient received a total of 80 mg of a drug in a 24 hour period. The suggested dosage range for the drug is between 0.01 g/kg per day and 0.015 g/kg per day. Is the amount of drug the patient received within the acceptable dosage range?

$\frac{75}{2.2} = 34.09 \text{ kg}$ $\frac{x \text{ mg}}{34.09 \text{ kg}} = \frac{10 \text{ mg}}{1 \text{ kg}}$

$x = 340.9 \text{ mg}$

$\frac{x \text{ mg}}{34.09 \text{ kg}} = \frac{15 \text{ mg}}{1 \text{ kg}}$

$x = 511.35 \text{ mg}$

YES or **(NO)**

The following problems require all of the skills that have been learned in the Dosage Calculations section.

32. A 56 kg patient is ordered to receive 1.5 mg/kg of a drug per dose. The drug is available as 100 mg/ml. How many ml are needed for one dose

$\frac{x \text{ mg}}{56 \text{ kg}} = \frac{1.5 \text{ mg}}{1 \text{ kg}}$ $\frac{x \text{ mL}}{84 \text{ mg}} = \frac{1 \text{ mL}}{100 \text{ mg}}$ $100x = 84$

$x = 84 \text{ mg/dose}$ $x = 0.84 \text{ mL}$

__0.84__ ml per dose

33. A physician has ordered that a 38 lb patient receive 0.25 mg/kg of a drug. The drug is available as 75 mg/3 ml. How many ml are needed?

$\frac{38}{2.2} = 17.27 \text{ kg}$ $\frac{x \text{ mg}}{17.27 \text{ kg}} = \frac{0.25 \text{ mg}}{1 \text{ kg}}$ $\frac{x \text{ mL}}{4.32 \text{ mg}} = \frac{3 \text{ mL}}{75 \text{ mg}}$ $75x = 12.96$

$x = 4.32 \text{ mg}$ $x = 0.173 \text{ mL}$

__0.173__ ml

Rx Success™ Complete Guide to Medical Math

34. A 150 lb patient is to receive 0.15 g/kg of a drug per day. The drug is available as 1.2 g/2 ml. How many ml are needed for one day?

$\frac{150}{2.2} = 68.18$ kg

$\frac{x\ g}{68.18\ kg} = \frac{0.15\ g}{1\ kg}$

$x = 10.23$ g/day

$\frac{x\ mL}{10.23\ g} = \frac{2\ mL}{1.2\ g}$

$1.2x = 20.46$
$x = 17.05$ mL

__17.05__ ml per day

35. The order reads: 2.4 mg/kg per dose. The patient weighs 130 lbs. How many ml are required when the drug is available in a concentration of 45 mg/ml?

$\frac{130}{2.2} = 59.09$ kg

$\frac{x\ mg}{59.09\ kg} = \frac{2.4\ mg}{1\ kg}$

$x = 141.82$ mg/dose

$\frac{x\ mL}{141.82\ mg} = \frac{1\ mL}{45\ mg}$

$45x = 141.82$
$x = 3.15$ mL

__3.15__ ml

36. A 65 lb patient is to receive 0.75 mg/kg per day in two equally divided doses. The drug is labeled as 15 mg/ml. How many ml are needed for one dose?

$\frac{65}{2.2} = 29.55$ kg

$\frac{x\ mg}{29.55\ kg} = \frac{0.75\ mg}{1\ kg}$

$x = 22.16$ mg/day / 2 = 11.08 mg/dose

$\frac{x\ mL}{11.08\ mg} = \frac{1\ mL}{15\ mg}$

$15x = 11.08$
$x = 0.74$ mL

__0.74__ ml per dose

37. The order reads: 0.02 g/kg per day in two equally divided doses. The patient weighs 74 lbs. The drug is available as 150 mg/ml. How many mls are needed per dose?

$\frac{74}{2.2} = 33.64$ kg

$\frac{x\ mg}{33.64\ kg} = \frac{20\ mg}{1\ kg}$

$x = 672.8$ mg/day / 2 = 336.4 mg/dose

$\frac{x\ mL}{336.4\ mg} = \frac{1\ mL}{150\ mg}$

$150x = 336.4$
$x = 2.24$ mL

__2.24__ ml per dose

38. A 36 lb patient is to receive 75 mcg/kg/day from a vial labeled 1.2 mg/2 ml. How many ml are needed for one day?

$\frac{36}{2.2} = 16.36$ kg

$\frac{x\ mg}{16.36\ kg} = \frac{0.075\ mg}{1\ kg}$

$x = 1.23$ mg/day

$\frac{x\ mL}{1.23\ mg} = \frac{2\ mL}{1.2\ mg}$

$1.2x = 2.46$
$x = 2.05$ mL/day

__2.05__ ml

Rx Success™ Complete Guide to Medical Math

39. The physician orders a 39 lb patient to receive 0.05 g per kg of body weight per day divided equally into 4 doses. The drug is available as 250 mg per 2 ml. How many ml will the patient receive in one dose?

$\frac{39}{2.2} = 17.73\ kg$ $\frac{X\ mg}{17.73\ kg} = \frac{50\ mg}{1\ kg}$

$X = 886.50\ mg/day\ /4 = 221.63\ mg/dose$

$\frac{X\ mL}{221.63\ mg} = \frac{2\ mL}{250\ mg}$ $250X = 443.26$ $X = 1.77\ mL$

__1.77__ ml

40. A 28 lb patient received 3.2 ml of a drug labeled as 0.05 mg per ml. The dosage range for this drug is between 15 mcg/kg and 25 mcg/kg. Is the amount of drug the patient received within the acceptable range?

$\frac{28}{2.2} = 12.73\ kg$ $\frac{X\ mg}{12.73\ kg} = \frac{0.015\ mg}{1\ kg}$ $X = 0.19\ mg$

$\frac{X\ mL}{0.19\ mg} = \frac{1\ mL}{0.05\ mg}$ $0.05X = 0.19$ $X = 3.8\ mL$

$\frac{X\ mg}{12.73\ kg} = \frac{0.025\ mg}{1\ kg}$ $X = 0.32\ mg$

$\frac{X\ mL}{0.32\ mg} = \frac{1\ mL}{0.05\ mg}$ $0.05X = 0.32$ $X = 6.4\ mL$

YES or **NO**

41. A 38 kg patient received a total of 50 ml of a drug labeled as 250 mg/5 ml, over a 5 day period of time. The dosage range for this drug is between 10 mg/kg per day and 20 mg/kg per day. Is the amount of drug the patient received within the acceptable range?

$\frac{X\ mg}{50\ mL} = \frac{250\ mg}{5\ mL}$ $5X = 12500$ $X = \frac{2500\ mg}{5} = 500\ mg/day$

$\frac{X\ mg}{38\ kg} = \frac{10\ mg}{1\ kg}$ $X = 380\ mg/day$

$\frac{X\ mg}{38\ kg} = \frac{20\ mg}{1\ kg}$ $X = 760\ mg/day$

YES or NO

42. A 112 kg patient received a dose of 1.25 ml of a drug labeled as 0.05 g/2.5 ml, three times per day. The dosage range for this drug is between 2.5 mg/kg per day and 4 mg/kg per day. Is the amount of drug the patient received within the acceptable range?

$\frac{X\ mg}{1.25\ mL} = \frac{50\ mg}{2.5\ mL}$ $2.5X = 62.5$ $X = 25\ mg/dose \times 3 = 75\ mg/day$

$\frac{X\ mg}{112\ kg} = \frac{2.5\ mg}{1\ kg}$ $X = 280\ mg/day$

$\frac{X\ mg}{112\ kg} = \frac{4\ mg}{1\ kg}$ $X = 448\ mg/day$

YES or **NO**

Rx Success™ Complete Guide to Medical Math

Chapter Ten

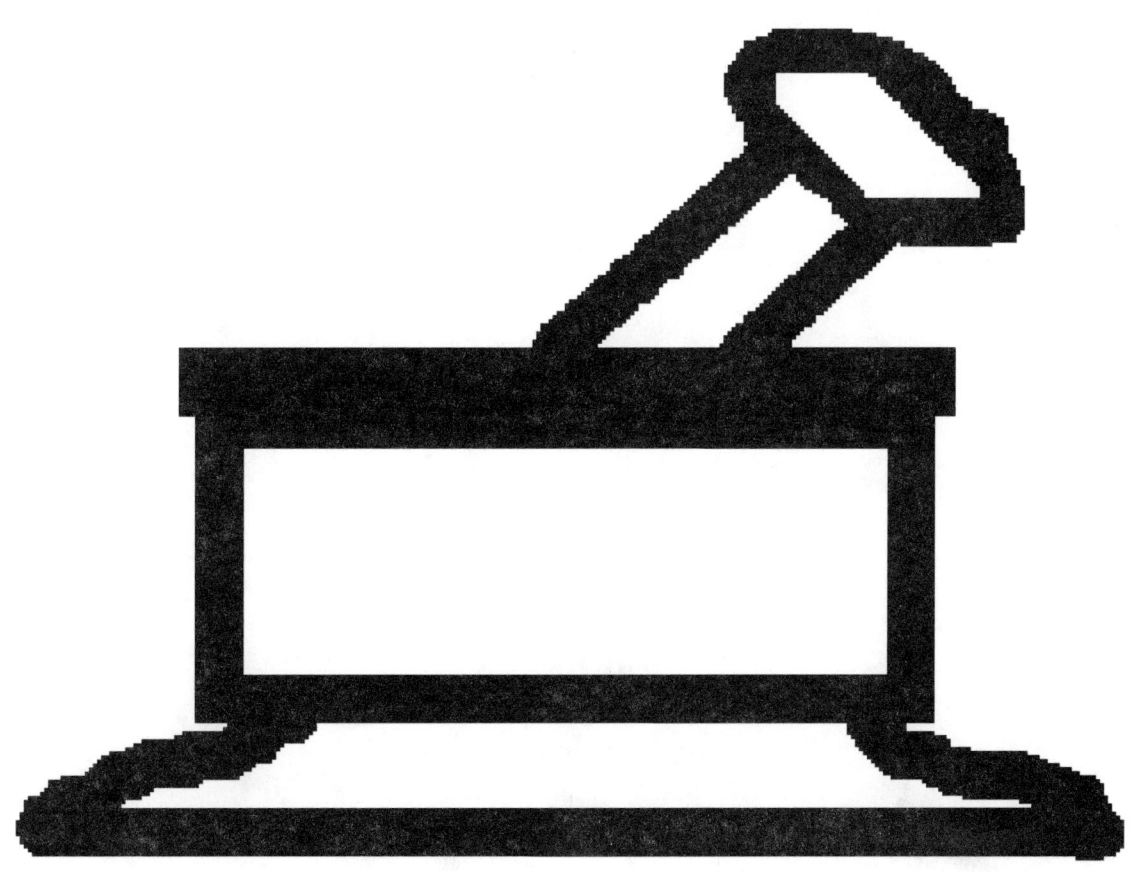

Insulin Calculations

Insulin Calculations

Insulin is used frequently, both in hospital settings and by many patients on an outpatient basis. There are many different types of insulin and each is used for very specific situations. It is important to understand these differences to ensure patient safety.

Historically, insulin has been harvested from the pancreas of cows (bovine insulin) and pigs (porcine insulin) and used successfully in humans. Most commonly used is a synthetically made human insulin. Porcine insulin differs from human insulin by only one amino acid (like all other proteins, insulin is made from strings of amino acids) and is chemically modified to make human insulin. Bovine insulin is no longer used because it is more antigenic (causes an immune response) than porcine or synthetic human insulin.

All insulin preparations are categorized based on three criteria:
- **Promptness** – How quickly does the insulin begin to work? You will see this value in the table under "Onset of Action" in the chart.
- **Intensity of Action** – When does the insulin reach its peak level of activity in the body? You will see this value under "Peak" in the chart.
- **Duration** – How long will the insulin work? You will see this value under "Duration of Action" in the chart.

The following table lists pharmacologic differences between the most commonly used types of insulin. Familiarize yourself with this table and the different types of insulin.

Type of Insulin	Onset of Action	Peak	Duration of Action
Insulin Aspart (Novolog®)	15 min	45 min	3-5 hours
Insulin Lispro (Humalog®)	0-15 min	30-90 min	6-8 hours
Regular Insulin	30-60 min	2.5-5 hours	6-8 hours
NPH Insulin	60-90 min	4-12 hours	24 hours
Lente® Insulin	1-2.5 hours	7-15 hours	24 hours
70/30 Insulin	30 min	4-8 hours	24 hours
Ultralente® Insulin	4-8 hours	16-18 hours	>36 hours
Insulin Glargine (Lantus®)	Constant, prolonged action over 24 hours, no pronounced peak		

Insulin is measured in units (like heparin), not milligrams or milliequivalents. The concentration (strength) of insulin that is used is...

100 U/1 ml

This strength is also referred to as "U-100". This means that for every one ml of insulin solution from the vial, there are exactly 100 units of actual insulin. Insulin syringes used by both patients and health care providers are based on U-100 insulin. These syringes are available in three different sizes.

Rx Success™ Complete Guide to Medical Math

- **30 Unit Syringe (1/3 cc)** – These syringes will accurately measure 30 units or less. The graphic below represents the markings on a 30 U insulin syringe. Note that each 5 U increment is represented by a number and each calibration (graduation marking) on the syringe represents one unit of insulin.

- **50 Unit Syringe (1/2 cc)** – Each 50 U syringe will accurately measure 50 units or less. Look at the graphic below to see the markings on a 50 U syringe. Like the 30 U syringe, each 5 U increment is represented by a number and each calibration (graduation marking) on the syringe represents one unit of insulin.

- **100 Unit Syringe (1 cc)** – A 100 U insulin syringe will accurately measure 100 units or less. Look at the graphic below to see the markings on a 100 U syringe. Each 10 U increment is represented by a number and each calibration (graduation marking) on the syringe represents *two units* of insulin.

Insulin Syringe Calibrations

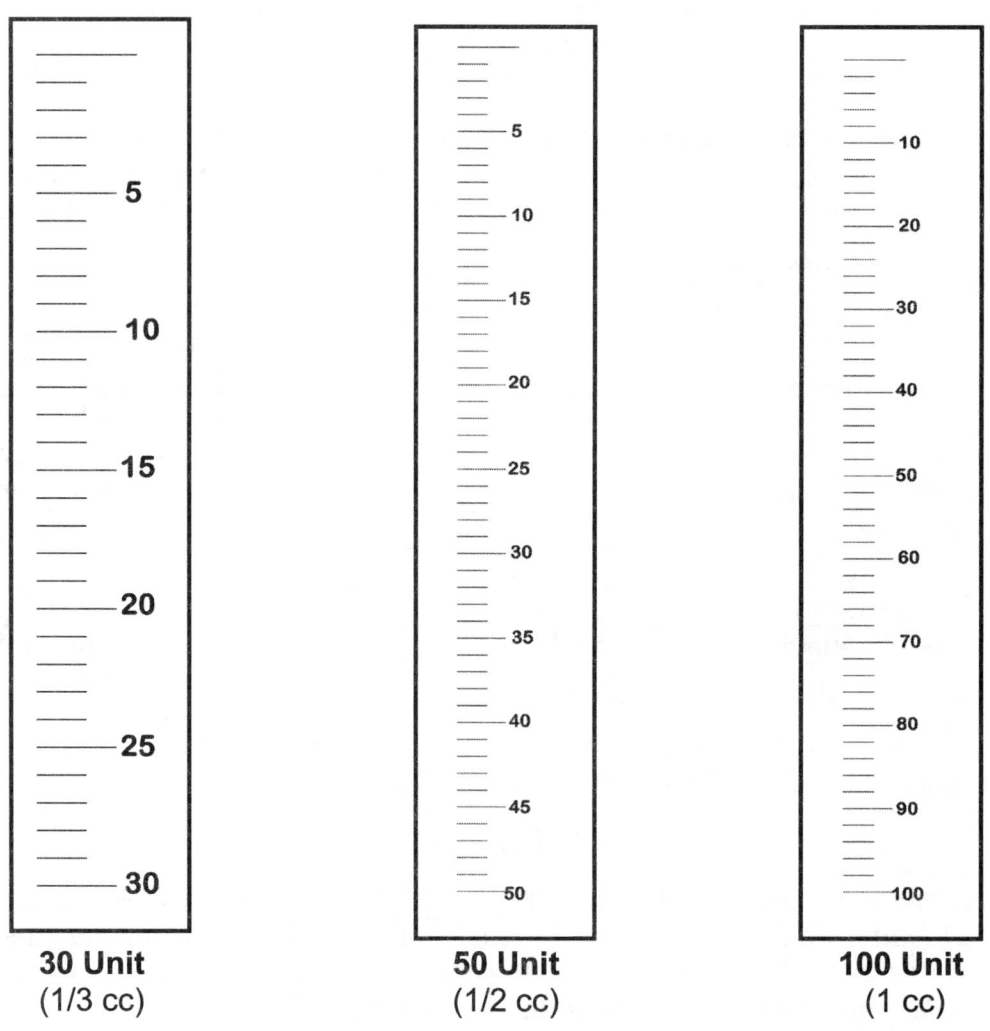

| 30 Unit | 50 Unit | 100 Unit |
| (1/3 cc) | (1/2 cc) | (1 cc) |

Rx Success™ Complete Guide to Medical Math

As with all injectable medications, use the smallest syringe available that will still hold the dose ordered. For instance:

Order	Syringe
17 units	30 Unit (1/3 cc)
43 units	50 unit (1/2 cc)
52 units	100 unit (1 cc)
37 units	50 unit (1/2 cc)
86 units	100 unit (1 cc)
7 units	30 unit (1/3 cc)

Combined Insulin Doses

Occasionally a patient needs more than one type of insulin throughout the day. Under these circumstances, it is common to combine two different types of insulin in the same syringe to reduce the number of injections for the patient. When combining insulins in a single syringe, remember:

- **When combining two insulins in the same syringe, the shortest acting insulin is *drawn up first!***

For instance, suppose a patient needs 10 U of Regular (R) insulin and 36 U of NPH insulin. The 10 U of Regular insulin would be drawn into the syringe first, followed by 36 U of NPH insulin, in the same syringe. Upon completion, the syringe plunger would be pulled back to a total of 46 U of insulin, preferably in a 50 U syringe.

Rx Success™ Complete Guide to Medical Math

Insulin Calculations - Sample Problems

Cross multiplication is used to calculate insulin doses, just like any other injectable medication. Here are some sample problems used for calculating insulin doses and determining the correct insulin syringe that should be used. **Assume that all insulin is U-100!**

1. **Order:** A patient is to receive 17 U of Regular, U-100 insulin. How many ml are needed for this dose? What size syringe should be used?

    100 units ⟷ 17 units
    1 ml ⟷ X ml

    $\frac{\cancel{100}X}{\cancel{100}} = \frac{17}{100}$

    X = 0.17ml   Using a 30 U syringe (1/3 cc).

2. A patient receives 0.32 ml of NPH, U-100 insulin. How many units of insulin did they receive?

    100 units ⟷ X units
    1 ml ⟷ 0.32 ml

    $\frac{\cancel{100}X}{\cancel{100}} = \frac{63}{100}$

    X = 32 U of insulin

3. **Order:** 26 units of Ultralente insulin, 17 units of Regular insulin. Which insulin should be drawn up first? What is the total volume in the syringe (how many ml)? What size syringe should be used?

    Step One: Looking at the insulin chart on page 151, we see that the Regular insulin is shorter acting than the Ultralente insulin. Therefore, the **Regular insulin should be drawn up first.**

Rx Success™ Complete Guide to Medical Math

Step Two: To determine the total volume in the syringe, we must determine the volume (number of ml) of each type of insulin and add them together.

$$\frac{100 \text{ units}}{1 \text{ ml}} = \frac{17 \text{ units}}{X \text{ ml}} \qquad\qquad \frac{100 \text{ units}}{1 \text{ ml}} = \frac{26 \text{ units}}{X \text{ ml}}$$

$$\frac{100x}{100} = \frac{17}{100} \qquad\qquad \frac{100X}{100} = \frac{26}{100}$$

$$X = 0.17 \text{ ml} \qquad\qquad X = 0.26 \text{ ml}$$

0.17 ml	+	0.26 ml	=	0.43 ml
Volume of Regular		**Volume of Ultralente**		**Total Volume**

Step Three: The possible choices for syringes are a 30 U (1/3 cc) syringe, a 50 U (1/2 cc) syringe and a 100 U (1 cc) syringe. Since we must use the smallest possible syringe that will hold the complete dose (0.43 ml), we will use the **50 U syringe (1/2 cc)**.

Rx Success™ Complete Guide to Medical Math

Insulin Calculations - Tutor Sheets™

USE THIS WORKSHEET AS A GUIDE TO HELP YOU SOLVE THE HOMEWORK PROBLEMS!

1. A patient is to receive 12 U of U-100 insulin. How many ml of U-100 insulin are needed for this dose?

   Code: 100 U = 1 ml

   $\dfrac{X\,mL}{12\,U} = \dfrac{1\,mL}{100\,U}$ $\quad 100X = 12$
   $\quad X = 0.12\,mL$

   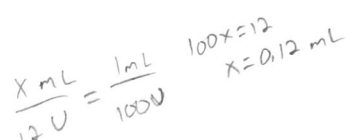

   $\dfrac{X\,mL}{12\,U} = \dfrac{1\,mL}{100\,U}$

   $100X = 12$

   $X = 0.12\,mL$

   _____ = _____

   X = __0.12__ ml

2. A patient is to receive 61 U of U-100 insulin. How many ml of U-100 insulin are needed for this dose?

   Code: _____ = _____

   $\dfrac{X\,mL}{61\,U} = \dfrac{1\,mL}{100\,U}$ $\quad 100X = 61$
   $\quad X = 0.61\,mL$

   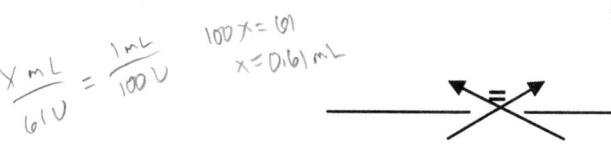

   _____ = _____

   X = __0.61__ ml

3. You are asked to compound a 2700 ml TPN for a patient containing 21 units of Regular insulin per liter of fluid. How many mls of U-100 insulin are needed?

   $\dfrac{X\,U}{2700\,mL} = \dfrac{21\,U}{1000\,mL}$ $\quad 1000X = 56700$
   $\quad X = 56.7\,U$

   $\dfrac{X\,mL}{56.7\,U} = \dfrac{1\,mL}{100\,U}$

   $X = 0.567\,mL$

   Step One: The order states that we need 21 units of insulin *per liter* of fluid. However, the total volume of the solution is given in *ml*. Therefore, the first step is to convert the volume of solution from *ml* to *liters*, using a metric conversion. For additional instruction on metric conversions please see **Chapter 5**.

   $\dfrac{X\,U}{2700\,mL} = \dfrac{21\,U}{1000\,mL}$

   $1000X = 56700$
   $X = 56.7\,U$

   $\dfrac{X\,mL}{56.7\,U} = \dfrac{1\,mL}{100\,U}$

   $100X = 56.7$
   $X = 0.567\,mL$

   2700 ml = __2.7__ L

Rx Success™ Complete Guide to Medical Math

Step Two: The order states that the IV solution is to contain 21 units of insulin per liter. Using the total number of liters of solution (found in step 1) and the order (21 U/1 L), calculate how many units of insulin are needed for the entire IV.

$$\frac{X \, U}{2.7 \, L} = \frac{21 \, U}{1 \, L}$$

$$X = 56.7 \, U$$

$$\frac{21 \, U}{1 \, L} \times = \times \frac{U}{L}$$

_____ = _____

X = _____ U

Step Three: Now that you have determined how many units of insulin are needed, you must use the concentration of the insulin (100 U/1 ml) to determine how many ml of insulin solution are needed.

Code: _____ U = _____ ml

$$\frac{X \, mL}{56.7 \, U} = \frac{1 \, mL}{100 \, U}$$

$$100X = 56.7$$
$$X = 0.567 \, mL$$

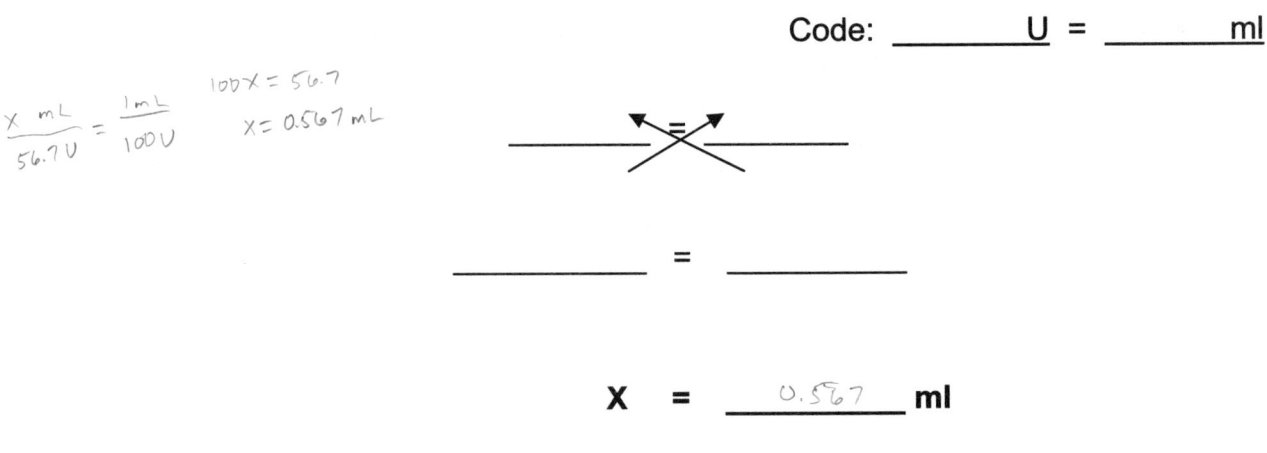

X = __0.567__ ml

---

4. You are asked to compound a 1250 ml TPN for a patient containing 32 units of Regular insulin per liter of fluid. How many mls of U-100 insulin are needed?

Step One: Convert the number of ml in the TPN into L using a metric conversion. For more information on Metric Conversions, see **Chapter 5**.

$$\frac{X \, U}{1250 \, mL} = \frac{32 \, U}{1000 \, mL}$$

$$1000X = 40000$$
$$X = 40 \, U$$

$$\frac{X \, mL}{40 \, U} = \frac{1 \, mL}{100 \, U}$$

$$100X = 40$$
$$X = 0.4 \, mL$$

1250 ml = _____ L

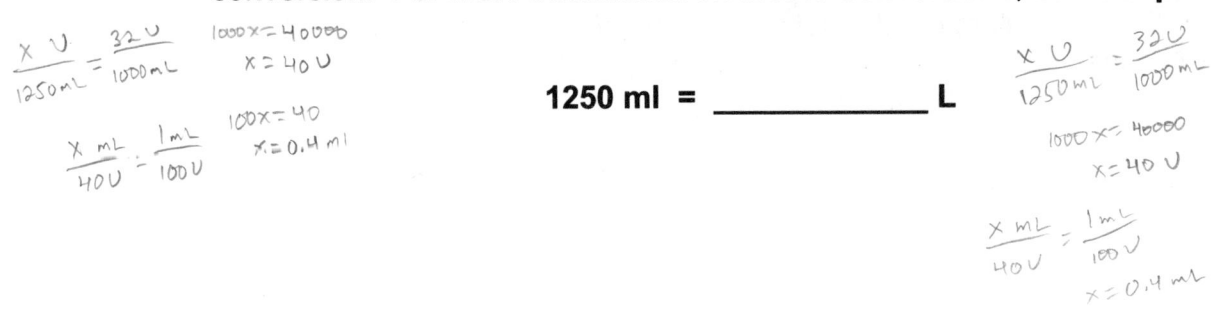

Rx Success™ Complete Guide to Medical Math

Step Two: Using the total number of liters of solution (found in step 1) and the order (32 U/1 L), calculate how many units of insulin are needed for the entire IV.

$$\frac{U}{L} = \frac{U}{L}$$

$$\underline{\qquad} = \underline{\qquad}$$

$$X = \underline{\qquad} U$$

Step Three: Now that you have determined how many units of insulin are needed, you must use the concentration of the insulin to determine how many ml of insulin solution are needed.

Code: _____ U = _____ ml

$$\underline{\qquad} = \underline{\qquad}$$

$$X = \underline{0.4}\ ml$$

---

5. **A patient is to receive 39 U of NPH insulin and 15 U of Regular insulin. Which insulin is drawn up first? What is the total volume of insulin in the syringe? What size syringe must be used?**

Step One: Which insulin is drawn up first? To determine which insulin is drawn up first, we must look at the insulin chart on page 125. Remember that *the shortest acting insulin is drawn up first!* When we compare NPH insulin and Regular insulin from the chart, we see that

_____Regular_____ insulin is drawn up first.

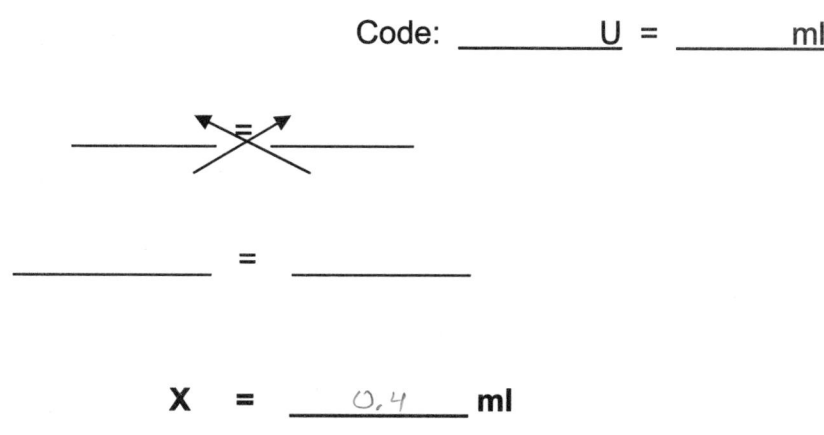

$39 + 15 = 54\ U$

$\dfrac{X\ mL}{54\ U} = \dfrac{1\ mL}{100\ U}$

$100x = 54$

$x = 0.54\ mL$

Page - 159

Rx Success™ Complete Guide to Medical Math

Step Two: What is the total volume of insulin in the syringe? Since there are two insulins that are being combined in the same syringe, we must calculate the volume of each insulin and add these volumes together. To perform this calculation, use the strength of the insulin (100 U/1 ml) as the code.

Volume of NPH insulin

$$\frac{100 \text{ U}}{1 \text{ ml}} = \frac{\underline{} \text{ U}}{X \text{ ml}}$$

_____ = _____

X = _____ ml

Volume of Regular Insulin

$$\frac{100 \text{ U}}{1 \text{ ml}} = \frac{\underline{} \text{ U}}{X \text{ ml}}$$

_____ = _____

X = _____ ml

Now, add the two volumes together to find the total volume!

_____ ml + _____ ml = __0.54__ ml
Volume of NPH   Volume of Regular   Total Volume

Step Three: Finally, we must determine which syringe to use. Remember that the correct syringe is the *smallest syringe that will hold the total volume!* There are three possible syringe sizes to choose from. Circle the best choice.

    1/3 cc   1/2 cc   **(1 cc)**

---

6. You are asked to simultaneously administer 12 U of Regular insulin and 32 U of Ultralente insulin, to a patient. Which insulin is drawn up first? What is the total volume of insulin in the syringe? What size syringe must be used?

Step One: Which insulin is drawn up first?

_____Regular_____ insulin is drawn up first.

12
32
44 U

$\frac{X \text{ mL}}{44 \text{ U}} = \frac{1 \text{ mL}}{100 \text{ U}}$

100x = 44
X = 0.44 mL

Rx Success™ Complete Guide to Medical Math

Step Two: What is the total volume of insulin in the syringe?

Volume of NPH insulin

```
_____ U=U _____ U
   ml              ml
```

_____ = _____

X = _____ ml

Volume of Regular Insulin

```
_____ U=U _____ U
   ml              ml
```

_____ = _____

X = _____ ml

Now, add the two volumes together to find the total volume!

_____ ml + _____ ml = ___0.44___ ml
Volume of Ultralente   Volume of Regular   Total Volume

Step Three: Determine which syringe to use. Circle the best choice.

1/3 cc   **(1/2 cc)**   **1 cc**

Answers to Tutor Sheets™ Calculations
1) 0.12 ml   2) 0.61 ml   3) 0.567 ml   4) 0.4 ml   5) Regular insulin; 0.54 ml; 1 cc
6) Regular insulin; 0.44 ml; 1/2 cc

Rx Success™ Complete Guide to Medical Math

Insulin Calculations - Homework

ASSUME WE ARE USING U-100 INSULIN
a. Calculate the following insulin doses.
b. Indicate what size insulin syringe will be used.

1. a. 26 units of insulin   =   __0.26__ ml

   $$\frac{26 \text{ units}}{x \, mL} = \frac{100 \text{ units}}{1 \, mL} \quad 100x = 26 \quad x = 0.26 \, mL \text{ or } cc$$

   b. Use a __1/3__ cc syringe.

2. a. 75 units of insulin   =   __0.75__ ml

   $$\frac{x \, mL}{75 \, U} = \frac{1 \, mL}{100 \, U} \quad 100x = 75 \quad x = 0.75 \, mL$$

   b. Use a __1__ cc syringe.

3. a. 14 units of insulin   =   __0.14__ ml

   $$\frac{x \, mL}{14 \, U} = \frac{1 \, mL}{100 \, U} \quad 100x = 14 \quad x = 0.14 \, mL$$

   b. Use a __1/3__ cc syringe.

4. a. 30 units of insulin   =   __0.30__ ml

   $$\frac{x \, mL}{30 \, U} = \frac{1 \, mL}{100 \, U} \quad 100x = 30 \quad x = 0.30 \, mL$$

   b. Use a __1/2__ cc syringe.

5. a. 7 units of insulin   =   __0.07__ ml

   $$\frac{x \, mL}{7 \, U} = \frac{1 \, mL}{100 \, U} \quad 100x = 7 \quad x = 0.07 \, mL$$

   b. Use a __1/3__ cc syringe.

6. a. 90 units of insulin   =   __0.9__ ml

   $$\frac{x \, mL}{90 \, U} = \frac{1 \, mL}{100 \, U} \quad 100x = 90 \quad x = 0.9 \, mL$$

   b. Use a __1__ cc syringe.

7. a. 54 units of insulin   =   __0.54__ ml

   $$\frac{x \, mL}{54} = \frac{1 \, mL}{100 \, U} \quad 100x = 54 \quad x = 0.54 \, mL$$

   b. Use a __1__ cc syringe.

Rx Success™ Complete Guide to Medical Math

8. **a.** 17 units of insulin = __0.17__ ml

   $\dfrac{X\,mL}{17\,U} = \dfrac{1\,mL}{100\,U}$ $100x = 17$ $x = 0.17\,mL$

   b. Use a __1/3__ cc syringe.

9. **a.** 34 units of insulin = __0.34__ ml

   $\dfrac{X\,mL}{34\,U} = \dfrac{1\,mL}{100\,U}$ $100x = 34$ $x = 0.34\,mL$

   b. Use a __1/2__ cc syringe.

10. **a.** 83 units of insulin = __0.83__ ml

    $\dfrac{X\,mL}{83\,U} = \dfrac{1\,mL}{100\,U}$ $100x = 83$ $x = 0.83\,mL$

    b. Use a __1__ cc syringe.

11. If a patient receives 0.6 ml of U-100 insulin, how many units of insulin did they receive?

    $\dfrac{X\,U}{0.6\,mL} = \dfrac{100\,U}{1\,mL}$ $x = 60\,U$

12. The patient is to receive 120 units of U-100 insulin in 1000 ml of NS, to be infused over 12 hours. To compound this IV, how many ml of U-100 insulin are needed?

    $\dfrac{X\,mL}{120\,U} = \dfrac{1\,mL}{100\,U}$ $100x = 120$ $x = 1.2\,mL$

13. A patient receives 0.15 ml of U-100 insulin, how many units of insulin did they receive?

    $\dfrac{X\,U}{0.15\,mL} = \dfrac{100\,U}{1\,mL}$ $x = 15\,U$

14. The physician's order states that the patient is to receive 35 U of Regular insulin three times daily. How many ml of insulin will be administered over four days?

    $\dfrac{X\,mL}{35\,U} = \dfrac{1\,mL}{100\,U}$ $100x = 35$ $x = 0.35\,mL \times 3 = 1.05\,mL/day \times 4 = 4.2\,mL$ total

Rx Success™ Complete Guide to Medical Math

15. You receive the following prescription: 32 U Regular insulin sq qd. How many ml of insulin does the patient need per dose?

    $$\frac{X\ mL}{32\ U} = \frac{1\ mL}{100\ U} \qquad 100x = 32 \qquad x = 0.32\ mL$$

16. A patient is to receive 75 units of insulin in 150 ml of NS via IV infusion. How many ml of U-100 insulin do you need to compound this IV?

    $$\frac{X\ mL}{75\ U} = \frac{1\ mL}{100\ U} \qquad 100x = 75 \qquad x = 0.75\ mL$$

    $$\frac{X\ mL}{75\ U} = \frac{1\ mL}{100\ U} \qquad 100x = 75 \qquad x = 0.75\ mL$$

17. You are asked to make a 3000 ml TPN for a patient. The TPN is to contain 16 units of U-100 insulin (regular) **per liter** of fluid. How many ml of U-100 insulin do you need?

    $$\frac{X\ U}{3000\ mL} = \frac{16\ U}{1000\ mL} \qquad 1000x = 48000 \qquad x = 48\ U$$

    $$\frac{X\ mL}{48\ U} = \frac{1\ mL}{100\ U} \qquad 100x = 48 \qquad x = 0.48\ mL$$

    $$\frac{X\ U}{3000\ mL} = \frac{16\ U}{1000\ mL} \qquad 1000x = 48000 \qquad x = 48\ U$$

    $$\frac{X\ mL}{48\ U} = \frac{1\ mL}{100\ U} \qquad x = 0.48\ mL$$

18. A patient is to receive 27 U of Regular insulin and 60 U of NPH insulin. Which insulin is drawn up first? What is the total volume of insulin in the syringe? What size syringe must be used?

    a) Insulin to be drawn up first? _____Regular_____

    b) Total volume of insulin in syringe? _____0.87 mL_____

    c) What size syringe? _____1 cc_____

19. A patient is to receive 47 U of NPH insulin and 20 U of Regular insulin. Which insulin is drawn up first? What is the total volume of insulin in the syringe? What size syringe must be used?

    a) Insulin to be drawn up first? _____Regular_____

    b) Total volume of insulin in syringe? _____0.67 mL_____

    c) What size syringe? _____1 cc_____

Rx Success™ Complete Guide to Medical Math

20. A patient is to receive 14 U of Regular insulin and 60 U of Lente insulin. Which insulin is drawn up first? What is the total volume of insulin in the syringe? What size syringe must be used?

    a) Insulin to be drawn up first? ___Regular___

    b) Total volume of insulin in syringe? __0.74 mL__

    c) What size syringe? ___1 cc___

21. A patient is to receive 33 U of Regular insulin and 52 U of NPH insulin. Which insulin is drawn up first? What is the total volume of insulin in the syringe? What size syringe must be used?

    a) Insulin to be drawn up first? ___Regular___

    b) Total volume of insulin in syringe? __0.85 mL__

    c) What size syringe? ___1 cc___

22. You are asked to make a 2700 ml TPN for a patient. The TPN is to contain 23 units of U-100 insulin (regular) **per liter** of fluid. How many ml of U-100 insulin do you need?

    $$\frac{X\ U}{2700\ mL} = \frac{23\ U}{1000\ mL} \qquad \frac{X\ mL}{62.1\ U} = \frac{1\ mL}{100\ mL}$$

    $1000 x = 62100 \qquad x = 0.621\ mL$

    $x = 62.1\ U$

23. You are asked to compound an intravenous solution containing 45 U of insulin in 375 ml of 0.9% saline. How many ml of U-100 insulin are needed to compound this IV?

    0.45 mL

Rx Success™ Complete Guide to Medical Math

24. While compounding a 3200 ml TPN for a patient, you add 1.6 ml of Regular insulin to the bag. The order said that the TPN was to contain 0.05 U of insulin per ml. Is the amount that you added to the TPN correct?

$$\frac{X\ U}{3200} = \frac{0.05\ U}{1\ mL}$$

$$x = 160\ U$$

$$\frac{X\ mL}{160\ U} = \frac{1\ mL}{100\ U}$$

$$100x = 160$$
$$x = 1.60\ mL$$

YES or NO

25. A patient receives two types of insulin in the same syringe. She needs 70 units of Ultralente insulin and 25 units of Regular insulin. Answer the following questions to prepare a dose for her.

   a) Which insulin must be drawn into the syringe first? Regular

   b) How many ml of Regular insulin are needed? 0.25 mL

   c) How many ml of Ultralente insulin are needed? 0.70 mL

   d) Which syringe should be used? 1 cc

Rx Success™ Complete Guide to Medical Math

Chapter Eleven

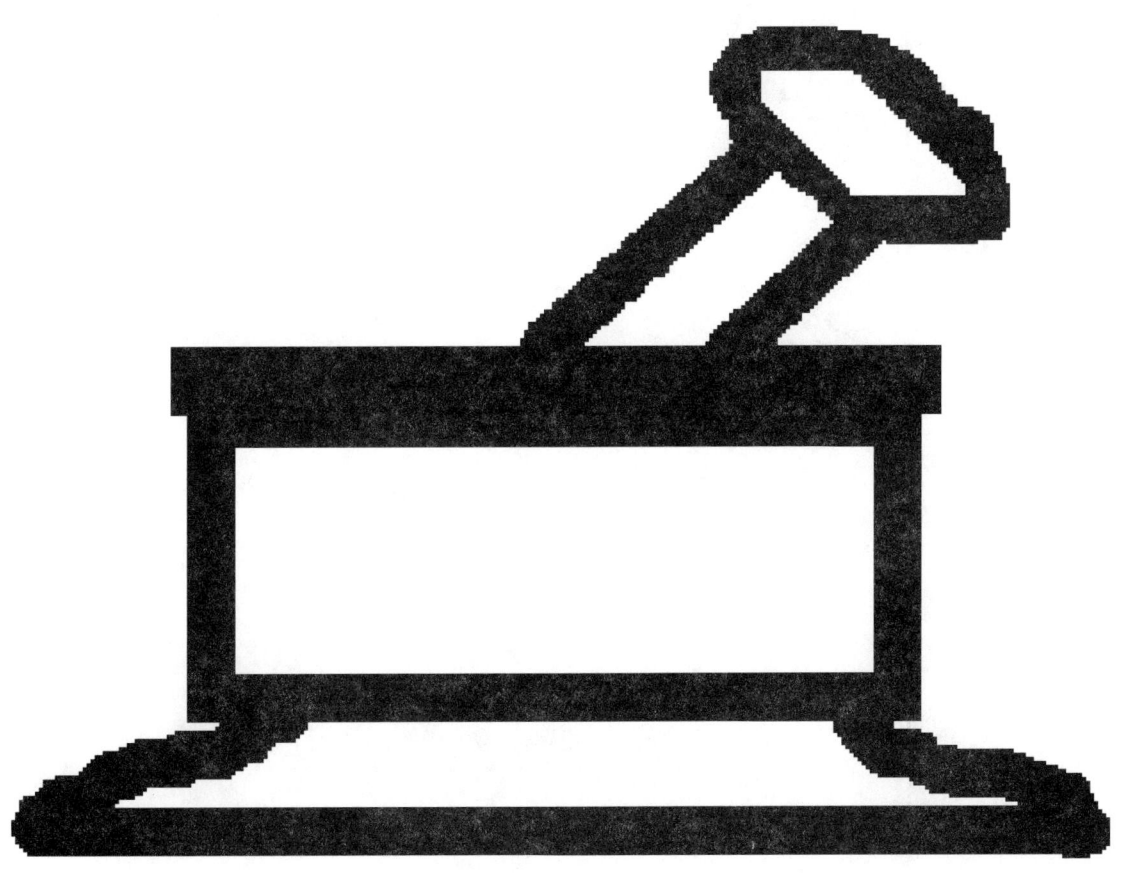

Percent Solutions

Rx Success™ Complete Guide to Medical Math

Rx Success™ Complete Guide to Medical Math

Percent Solutions

Often, health care providers come into contact with medications whose strengths are expressed as percentages. These compounds are called *percent solutions* and are generally creams, ointments or liquid solutions. Percent solutions are commonly made by mixing a **solute** (aka *active ingredient* or *drug*) with some sort of **vehicle**. For example, D_5W, one of the most prevalently used IV solutions, stands for 5% Dextrose in Water. In this case, dextrose is the solute which has been dissolved in a vehicle (water). The percent strength (5%) simply refers to how much dextrose has been dissolved into the vehicle.

The term "percent", when dealing with solutions, means grams of solute per 100 parts of the total compound. The percent strength of the solution *always* refers to the amount of solute (drug) in the solution, *not* the amount of vehicle. D5W, contains 5 grams of Dextrose per 100 ml of solution (5 g/100 ml). A 34% Saline solution will contain 34 grams of salt per 100 ml of solution (34 g/100 ml).

The most important thing to do when you encounter a percent solution is to first…

CONVERT THE PERCENT STRENGTH TO A FRACTION WITH UNITS!

Percents are very difficult to work with by themselves; however, when converted to a fraction, the percent strength of a solution can be used as a conversion factor for a cross multiplication problem. Once the percent strength is converted to a fraction, the fraction denotes how much total drug is present in a particular amount of the entire solution. For instance, in a 70% liquid solution, there are 70 grams of drug per every 100 mls of solution (70 g/100 ml).

70% Solution   means   **70 g of Drug per 100 ml of Solution**

When working with percent solutions, there are two types that are most commonly used. One type of percent solution is in liquid form and the other is in solid form.

Liquid Percent Solutions: These percent solutions are easy to spot because they are always liquids and they are always measured in liquid volume units like ml or L. To convert liquid percent solutions to a fraction, simply replace the "%" sign with "g" and place the remaining number over "100 ml". For instance, a 1.5% solution becomes 1.5 g/100 ml. This means that if you were to pour out 100 ml from that bottle of 1.5% solution, there would be exactly 1.5 g of drug in that 100 ml.

1.5% Solution   means   **1.5 g of Drug per 100 ml of Solution**

Example: Create a fraction from this bottle of a liquid, percent solution preparation.

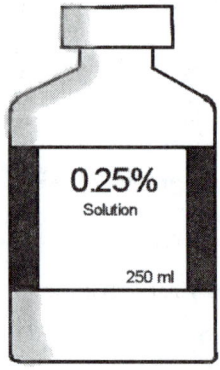

The percent strength on this bottle is **0.25%**. First, remove the the "%" sign and replace with the unit, "grams". Then, place the remaining number over "100 mls". The final fraction is

<u>**0.25 grams**</u>
100 mls

This fraction literally means that every 100 mls of solution poured out of this bottle contains 0.25 grams of pure drug. The remainder of the 100 ml of solution is considered to be part of the vehicle.

Solid Percent Solutions: These are percent solutions that *cannot* be measured in mls. These are preparations like creams or ointments, which are measured in grams. To convert these percent strengths into a fraction, remove the "%" sign and replace with "grams of drug". Then, place this number over "100 grams of cream (or ointment)".

Example: Create a fraction from this tube of a solid, percent solution preparation.

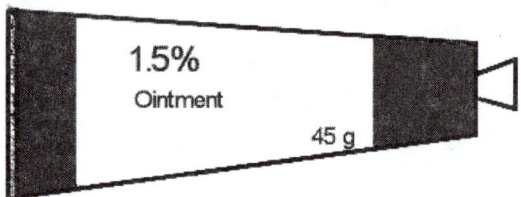

The percent strength on this tube of ointment is **1.5%**. First, remove the "%" sign and replace with the unit, "grams of drug". Then, place the remaining number over "100 g of ointment". The final fraction is

<u>**1.5 g of drug**</u>
100 g of ointment

This fraction literally means that for every 100 grams of this 1.5% ointment, there are exactly 1.5 grams of pure drug.

The following table contains several different types of percent solutions in both liquid and solid forms. The second column denotes how many grams of drug are in 100 parts of each percent solution. The final column lists the correct fractions, with units, for each of the percent solutions.

Rx Success™ Complete Guide to Medical Math

Percent Solution	Grams per 100 parts	Fraction with Units
Normal Saline (0.9%)	0.9	**0.9 g/100 ml**
Dextrose 5% in Water	5	**5 g/100 ml**
½ Normal Saline (0.45%)	0.45	**0.45 g/100 ml**
70% Dextrose in Water	70	**70 g/100 ml**
¼ Normal Saline (0.225%)	0.225	**0.225 g/100 ml**
1% Clobetasol Ointment	1	**1 g drug/100 g oint**
2.5% Triamcinolone Cream	2.5	**2.5 g drug/100 g crm**

One type of calculation that can be performed, with these fractions, is to determine how much drug (or solute) is in any amount of the solution. These fractions will also allow you to determine how many grams of a particular drug are needed *to make* any amount of a percent solution.

Study the Sample Problems that follow and then complete the Tutor Sheets™. Finally, complete the Percent Solution Homework at the end of the chapter to master Percent Solution calculations.

Rx Success™ Complete Guide to Medical Math
Percent Solutions - Sample Problems

1. How many grams of drug are in 450 ml of a 25% solution?

We know that a 25% solution contains 25 grams of drug per 100 ml of solution. Set up the cross multiplication problem like this:

$$\frac{25 \text{ grams drug}}{100 \text{ ml}} = \frac{X \text{ grams drug}}{450 \text{ ml}}$$

$$\frac{25 \text{ grams drug}}{100 \text{ ml}} \times\!\!=\!\!\times \frac{X \text{ grams drug}}{450 \text{ ml}}$$

$$\frac{\cancel{100}\,X}{\cancel{100}} = \frac{11{,}250}{100}$$

$$X = 112.5 \text{ grams}$$

Handwritten work:
$\frac{X\,g}{450\,mL} = \frac{25\,g}{100\,mL}$ $100X = 11250$ $X = 112.50 \text{ grams}$

---

2. How many grams of drug are in 515 ml of a 0.225% solution?

We know that a 0.225% solution contains 0.225 grams of drug per 100 ml of solution. Set up the cross multiplication problem like this:

$$\frac{0.225 \text{ grams drug}}{100 \text{ ml}} = \frac{X \text{ grams drug}}{515 \text{ ml}}$$

$$\frac{0.225 \text{ grams drug}}{100 \text{ ml}} \times\!\!=\!\!\times \frac{X \text{ grams drug}}{515 \text{ ml}}$$

$$\frac{\cancel{100}\,X}{\cancel{100}} = \frac{115.88}{100}$$

$$X = 1.16 \text{ grams}$$

Handwritten work:
$\frac{X\,g}{515\,mL} = \frac{0.225\,g}{100\,mL}$ $100X = 115.88$ $X = 1.16\,g$

---

3. How many grams of a 1.5% cream can be made with 5 grams of hydrocortisone powder?

Handwritten work:
$\frac{X\,g}{5\,g} = \frac{100\,g}{1.5\,g}$ $1.5X = 500$ $X = 333.33\,g \text{ crm}$

a) As with all other percent solution problems, convert the "1.5%" into a fraction with units and then use that fraction as the code to determine how many grams of cream you could make with 5 grams of drug.

Page - 175

Rx Success™ Complete Guide to Medical Math

$$\frac{1.5 \text{ g drug}}{100 \text{ g crm}} = \frac{5 \text{ g drug}}{X \text{ g crm}}$$

b) The final step is to cross multiply.

$$\frac{1.5 \text{ g drug}}{100 \text{ g crm}} \diagup\!\!\!= \frac{5 \text{ g drug}}{X \text{ g crm}}$$

$$\frac{\cancel{1.5}X}{\cancel{1.5}} = \frac{500}{1.5}$$

$$X = 333.33$$

A total of **333.33 grams of cream** could be made.

---

4. **Calculate the percent strength when 2.5 grams of drug is dissolved in 1250 ml of solution?**

   We know that the percent strength for a liquid drug *must* be in this format

   [handwritten: $\frac{X g}{100 mL} = \frac{2.5 g}{1250 mL}$ $1250X = 250$ $X = 0.2 g$ or 0.2%]

   $$\frac{\text{g drug}}{100 \text{ ml}}$$

   Furthermore, we know that whatever number is in the numerator of this fraction IS the percent strength! To solve this problem, take the information given in the problem and convert it to the format of the above fraction. The cross multiplication problem is set up this way.

   [handwritten: $\frac{X g}{100 mL} = \frac{2.5 g}{1250 mL}$ $1250X = 250$ $x = 0.2 g$ or 0.2%]

   $$\frac{2.5 \text{ g drug}}{1250 \text{ ml soln}} = \frac{X \text{ g drug}}{100 \text{ ml soln}}$$

   $$0.2 = X$$

   When the problem is solved we find that there are 0.2 grams of drug in every 100 ml of solution.

   $$\frac{0.2 \text{ g drug}}{100 \text{ ml}}$$

Now that the fraction is in the proper format, simply take the number in the numerator position (0.2) and this is percent strength. The final answer is **0.2%.**

Rx Success™ Complete Guide to Medical Math

Percent Solutions – Tutor Sheets™

USE THIS WORKSHEET AS A GUIDE TO HELP YOU SOLVE THE HOMEWORK PROBLEMS!

1. How many grams of drug are in 850 ml of a 0.25% solution?

    Step One: Convert the percent strength to a fraction with units!

    $$\frac{\text{___ g drug}}{100 \text{ ml soln}}$$

    (handwritten):
    $$\frac{X \text{ g}}{850 \text{ mL}} = \frac{0.25 \text{ g}}{100 \text{ mL}}$$
    $$100X = 212.50$$
    $$X = 2.13 \text{ g}$$

    Step Two: Use the fraction with units as the code to set up a cross multiplication problem. This calculation will provide the number of grams of drug in 850 ml of the 0.25% solution.

    $$\frac{\text{___ g drug}}{\text{___ ml soln}} = \frac{X \text{ g drug}}{\text{___ ml soln}}$$

    (handwritten):
    $$\frac{X \text{ g}}{850 \text{ mL}} = \frac{0.25 \text{ g}}{100 \text{ mL}}$$
    $$100X = 212.5$$
    $$X = 2.13 \text{ g}$$

    Cross multiply…

    $$\frac{\text{___ g drug}}{\text{___ ml soln}} \diagup\!\!\!= \frac{X \text{ g drug}}{\text{___ ml soln}}$$

    $$\text{_____} = 100X$$

    $$\text{_____} = X$$

---

2. How many grams of a 0.225% cream can be made with 0.75 g of drug?

    Step One: Convert the percent strength to a fraction with units!

    (handwritten left):
    $$\frac{X \text{ g crm}}{0.75 \text{ g}} = \frac{100 \text{ g crm}}{0.225 \text{ g}}$$
    $$0.225X = 75$$
    $$X = 333.33 \text{ g of crm}$$

    $$\frac{\text{___ g drug}}{100 \text{ g crm}}$$

    (handwritten right):
    $$\frac{X \text{ g crm}}{0.75 \text{ g}} = \frac{100 \text{ g crm}}{0.225 \text{ g}}$$
    $$0.225X = 75$$
    $$X = 333.33 \text{ g crm}$$

    Step Two: Use the fraction with units as the code to set up a cross multiplication problem. This calculation will provide the number of grams of 0.225% cream that can be made with 0.75 g of drug.

    $$\frac{\text{___ g drug}}{\text{___ g crm}} = \frac{\text{___ g drug}}{\text{___ g crm}}$$

Rx Success™ Complete Guide to Medical Math

Cross multiply...

$$\frac{\text{g drug}}{\text{g crm}} \diagup= \diagup \frac{\text{g drug}}{\text{g crm}}$$

X = _____

X = _____

---

3. How many grams of a 0.5% ointment can be made with 1200 mg of drug?

Step One: Convert the percent strength to a fraction with units!

$$\frac{\text{g drug}}{100 \text{ g oint}}$$

Handwritten:
$$\frac{X \text{ g oint}}{1.2 \text{ g}} = \frac{100 \text{ g oint}}{0.5 \text{ g}}$$
$$0.5x = 120$$
$$x = 240 \text{ g oint}$$

Step Two: Use the fraction with units as the code to set up a cross multiplication problem. However, notice that the amount of drug we have (1200 mg) is in **mg** yet our cross multiplication problem is in **gram** units. Therefore, we must first convert the amount of drug that we have into grams (remember Metric Conversions!).

Handwritten:
$$\frac{X \text{ g oint}}{1.2 \text{ g}} = \frac{100 \text{ g oint}}{0.5 \text{ g}}$$
$$0.5x = 120$$
$$x = 240 \text{ g oint}$$

1200 mg = _____ g

Now you can set up a cross multiplication problem that will provide the number of grams of 0.5% ointment that can be made with 1.2 g of drug.

$$\frac{\text{g drug}}{\text{g oint}} = \frac{\text{g drug}}{\text{g oint}}$$

Cross multiply...

$$\frac{\text{g drug}}{\text{g oint}} \diagup= \diagup \frac{\text{g drug}}{\text{g oint}}$$

X = _____

Rx Success™ Complete Guide to Medical Math

X = _____

---

4. Calculate the percent strength of 1.2 L of solution that contains 12 g of drug.

   We know that the percent strength for a liquid drug *must* be in this format

   g drug
   100 ml

   $$\frac{12\,g}{1200\,mL} = \frac{x\,g}{100\,mL}$$
   $$1200x = 1200$$
   $$x = 1\,g$$
   or 1%.

   Furthermore, we know that whatever number is in the numerator of this fraction IS the percent strength! To solve this problem, we will take the information given in the problem and convert it to the format of the above fraction.

   Notice that the format we *want* has the volume units of the solution listed as **ml**, yet in the problem, the volume units are listed as **Liters**. Therefore the very first step is to convert the volume units of our problem into ml.

   1.2 L = _____ ml

   $$\frac{12\,g}{1200\,mL} = \frac{x\,g}{100\,mL}$$
   $$1200 = 1200x$$
   $$x = 1\,g \text{ or } 1\%$$

   And now, we are able to set up the cross multiplication problem.

   $$\frac{g\ drug}{ml\ soln} = \frac{X\ g\ drug}{100\ ml\ soln}$$

   X = _____

   X = _____

   Now that we know how many g of drug are in 100 ml of this solution, simply add a percent sign and the final answer is

   _____ %

Answers to Tutor Sheets™ Calculations
1) 2.13 g   2) 333.33 g   3) 240 g   4) 1%

Rx Success™ Complete Guide to Medical Math

Percent Solutions - Homework

Calculate the following problems using the percents given.

1. How many grams of drug are in 200 ml of a 1.5% solution?

    $$\frac{x\,g}{200\,mL} = \frac{1.5\,g}{100\,mL} \qquad 100x = 300 \\ x = 3\,g$$

2. How many grams of drug are in 375 ml of a 3% solution?   *3 g*

    $$\frac{x\,g}{375\,mL} = \frac{3\,g}{100\,mL} \qquad 100x = 1125 \\ x = 11.25\,g$$

3. How many grams of drug are in 1500 ml of a 0.5% solution?   *11.25 g*

    $$\frac{x\,g}{1500\,mL} = \frac{0.5\,g}{100\,mL} \qquad 100x = 750 \\ x = 7.5\,g$$

4. How many grams of drug are in 150 ml of a 3.75% solution?   *7.5 g*

    $$\frac{x\,g}{150\,mL} = \frac{3.75\,g}{100\,mL} \qquad 100x = 562.5 \\ x = 5.625\,g$$

5. How many grams of drug are in 1250 ml of a 12% solution?   *5.63 g*

    $$\frac{x\,g}{1250\,mL} = \frac{12\,g}{100\,mL} \qquad 100x = 15000 \\ x = 150\,g$$

6. How many grams of drug are in 850 ml of a 70% solution?   *150 g*

    $$\frac{x\,g}{850\,mL} = \frac{70\,g}{100\,mL} \qquad 100x = 59500 \\ x = 595\,g$$

7. How many grams of drug are in 25 ml of a 10% solution?   *595 g*

    $$\frac{x\,g}{25\,mL} = \frac{10\,g}{100\,mL} \qquad 100x = 250 \\ x = 2.5\,g$$

2.5 g

Rx Success™ Complete Guide to Medical Math

8. How many grams of drug are in 500 ml of a 0.225% solution? 1.13 g

$$\frac{x\,g}{500\,mL} = \frac{0.225\,g}{100\,mL}$$
$$100x = 112.5$$
$$x = 1.13\,g$$

9. How many grams of drug are in 1050 ml of a 0.15% solution? 1.58 g

$$\frac{x\,g}{1050\,mL} = \frac{0.15\,g}{100\,mL}$$
$$100x = 157.5$$
$$x = 1.58\,g$$

10. How many grams of drug are in 75 ml of a 2.5% solution? 1.88 g

$$\frac{x\,g}{75\,mL} = \frac{2.5\,g}{100\,mL} \quad 100x = 187.5$$
$$x = 1.88\,g$$

11. How many ml of 0.25% solution can be made with 1 Liter of a 1.5% solution? 6000 mL

$$\frac{x\,g}{1000\,mL} = \frac{1.5\,g}{100\,mL}$$
$$100x = 1500$$
$$x = 15\,g$$

$$\frac{x\,mL}{15\,g} = \frac{100\,mL}{0.25\,g}$$
$$0.25x = 1500$$
$$x = 6000\,mL$$

$$\frac{x\,mL}{15\,g} = \frac{100\,mL}{0.25\,g} \quad 0.25x = 1500$$
$$x = 6000\,mL$$

$$\frac{y\,g}{1000\,mL} = \frac{1.5\,g}{100\,mL} \quad 100x = 1500$$
$$x = 15\,g$$

12. How many grams of a 35% cream can be made with 1 lb of a 42% cream? 544.8 g

$$\frac{x\,kg}{1\,lb} = \frac{1\,kg}{2.2\,lb} \quad 2.2x = 1$$
$$x = 0.45\,kg$$

$$\frac{x\,g}{454\,g\,crm} = \frac{42\,g}{100\,g\,crm} \quad 100x = 19068$$
$$x = 190.68\,g$$

$$\frac{x\,g\,crm}{190.68\,g} = \frac{100\,g\,crm}{35\,g} \quad 35x = 19068$$
$$x = 544.8\,g\,crm$$

$$\frac{x\,kg}{1\,lb} = \frac{1\,kg}{2.2\,lb} \quad 2.2x = 1 \quad x = 0.45\,kg$$
$$\frac{x\,g}{450\,g\,crm} = \frac{42\,g}{100\,g\,crm} \quad 100x = 18900 \quad x = 189\,g$$
$$\frac{x\,g\,crm}{189\,g} = \frac{100\,g\,crm}{35\,g} \quad 35x = 18900 \quad x = 540\,g\,crm$$

13. You have 2.5 L of a 5% ascorbic acid solution. How many FULL, 150 ml bottles of 2.5% ascorbic acid solution can you make? 33 full bottles

$$\frac{x\,g}{2500\,mL} = \frac{5}{100\,mL}$$
$$100x = 12500$$
$$x = 125\,g$$

$$\frac{x\,mL}{125\,g} = \frac{100\,mL}{2.5\,g}$$
$$2.5x = 12500$$
$$x = 5000\,mL/150\,mL = 33\,full\,150\,mL\,bottles$$

$$\frac{x\,g}{2500\,mL} = \frac{5}{100\,mL} \quad 100x = 12500 \quad x = 125\,g$$
$$\frac{x\,mL}{125\,g} = \frac{100\,mL}{2.5\,g} \quad 2.5x = 12500 \quad x = 5000\,mL/150 = 33\,bottles$$

14. A 250 ml bottle contains 7.5 grams of a drug. Calculate the percent strength of this solution. 3%

$$\frac{x\,g}{100\,mL} = \frac{7.5\,g}{250\,mL} \quad 250x = 750$$
$$x = 3 \text{ or } 3\%$$

$$\frac{7.5\,g}{250\,mL} = \frac{x\,g}{100\,mL}$$
$$250x = 750$$
$$x = 3\,g \text{ or } 3\%$$

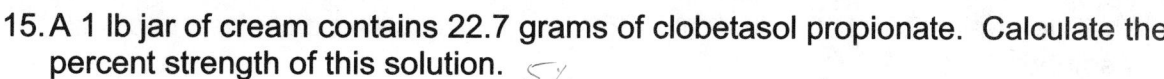

15. A 1 lb jar of cream contains 22.7 grams of clobetasol propionate. Calculate the percent strength of this solution. 5%

16. A 45 g tube of ointment contains 1,125 mg of hydrocortisone. Calculate the percent strength of this tube of ointment. 2.5%

17. A 3 L bag of 0.5% irrigation solution, contains how many grams of drug? 15 g

18. Calculate the percent strength of a dextrose solution containing a total of 2.3 L of solution and 115,000 mg of dextrose. 5%

19. How many grams of a 0.25% hydrocortisone cream can be made with 1.5 lbs of a 4% hydrocortisone cream? 10896 g

20. Calculate the percent strength when 50 grams of drug is dissolved into 500 mls of solution. 10%

21. Calculate the percent strength when 15 grams of drug is dissolved into 750 mls of solution. 2%

22. What percent strength results from 1250 mg of drug being dissolved into 3.75 L of solution? 0.03%

$$\frac{x\,g}{100\,mL} = \frac{1.25\,g}{3750\,mL} \quad 3750x = 125 \quad x = 0.03\,g \text{ or } 0.03\%$$

$$\frac{x\,g}{100\,mL} = \frac{1.25\,g}{3750\,mL}$$
$$3750x = 125$$
$$x = 0.03\,g \text{ or } 0.03\%$$

23. A 2.3 L bag of NS contains 0.25 g of drug per Liter of solution. Calculate the percent strength of this solution. 0.025%

$$\frac{x\,g}{2.3\,L} = \frac{0.25\,g}{1\,L} \quad x = 0.575\,g$$

$$\frac{x\,g}{100\,mL} = \frac{0.575\,g}{2300\,mL} \quad 2300x = 57.5 \quad x = 0.025\,g \text{ or } 0.025\%$$

$$\frac{x\,g}{2300\,mL} = \frac{0.25\,g}{1000\,mL} \quad 1000x = 575 \quad x = 0.575\,g$$

$$\frac{x\,g}{100\,mL} = \frac{0.575\,g}{2300\,mL} \quad 2300x = 57.5 \quad x = 0.025\,g \text{ or } 0.025\%$$

24. A 1.5 L bag of Dextrose solution contains 5 mg/ml of a drug. Calculate the percent strength of this solution. 0.5%

$$\frac{x\,g}{1500\,mL} = \frac{0.005\,g}{1\,mL} \quad x = 7.5\,g$$

$$\frac{x\,g}{100\,mL} = \frac{7.5\,g}{1500\,mL} \quad 1500x = 750 \quad x = 0.5\,g \text{ or } 0.5\%$$

$$\frac{x\,g}{1500\,mL} = \frac{0.005\,g}{1\,mL} \quad x = 7.5\,g$$

$$\frac{x\,g}{100\,mL} = \frac{7.5\,g}{1500\,mL} \quad 1500x = 750 \quad x = 0.5\,g \text{ or } 0.5\%$$

Rx Success™ Complete Guide to Medical Math

Chapter Twelve

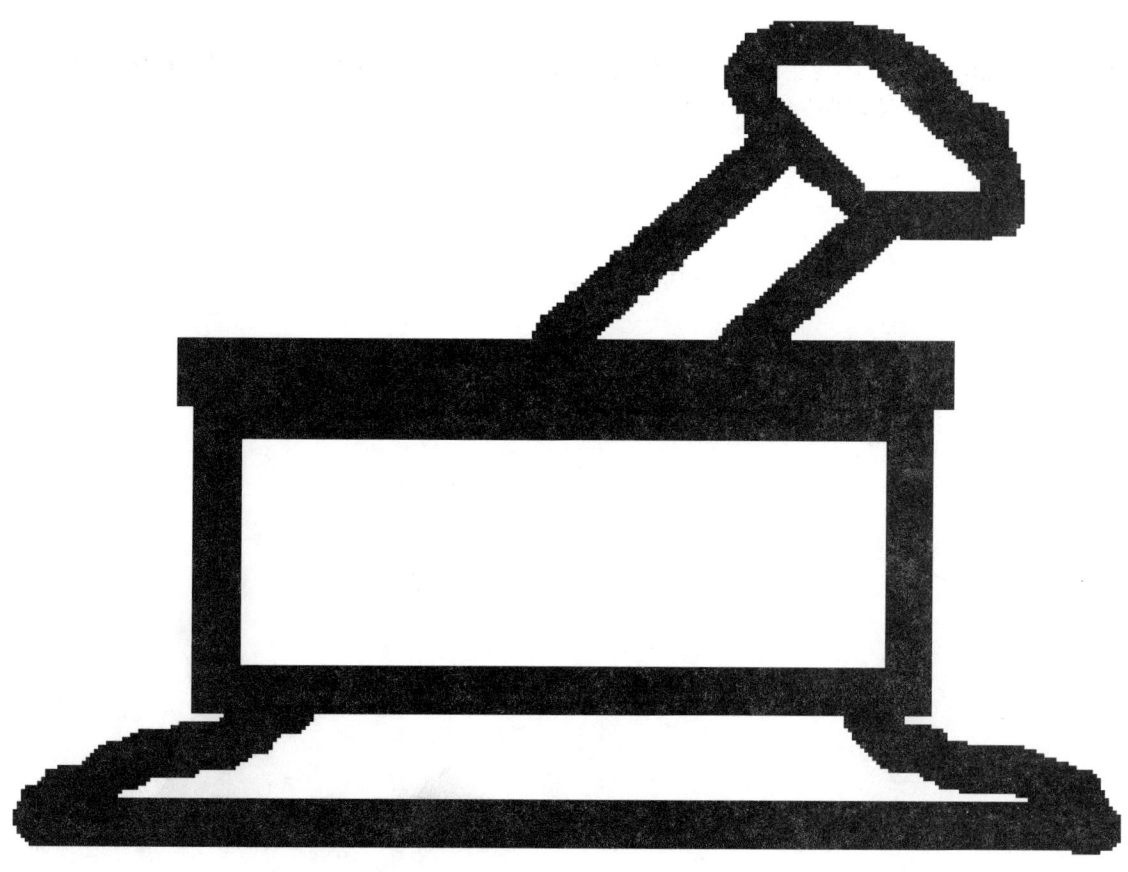

IV Drip Rate Calculations

IV Solutions

Before beginning a discussion of IV Drip Rate Calculations, it is important to have a basic understanding of common IV solutions that are used as vehicles for medications. IV drugs are usually added to bags of fluid for direct infusion into the body. The fluid in these bags must not only be compatible with the body but also the drug. If an IV must be compounded, the medication order will list the name of the drug, the amount of drug and also the correct IV fluid with which to mix the drug.

There are several different types of IV solutions that are compatible with the body when given intravenously. Bags of these common fluids come in many different sizes and fluid combinations. Because these solutions are compatible with the body, they can be used as vehicles to deliver drug into the body (with the exception of Sterile Water for Injection – Large volumes of SWFI are *not* used for direct IV infusion.). Here are the most commonly used IV solutions.

1. **Dextrose Solutions** – The body runs on a sugar fuel called glucose. Dextrose is a sugar that is structurally very similar to glucose. The body can use dextrose just as readily as it can use glucose, making a dextrose solution very compatible with the body. Dextrose solutions can be used to treat hypoglycemia (glucose deficiency in the blood) or as a fluid replacement solution. Because of the sugar content, dextrose solutions must be used with caution in diabetic patients. There are several different strengths of dextrose solutions that are commercially available.

   - D5W (5% Dextrose in Water)
   - D10W (10% Dextrose in Water)
   - D50 (50% Dextrose in Water)
   - D70 (70% Dextrose in Water)

2. **Saline Solutions** – The word saline simply refers to a solution that contains the salt, sodium chloride (table salt). Normal saline is the most commonly used IV saline solution. It is called "Normal Saline", or NS, because the salt concentration in the solution exactly matches the salt concentration in the cells of the body. This equivalent concentration is referred to as "isotonic" and has a concentration of 0.9% saline. Like all percent solutions, the percentage refers to the amount of salt (or drug) in grams, per 100 mls of solution. Saline solutions can be used for fluid

replacement or to restore sodium and/or chlorine ion balance in the body. There are also saline solutions that are *less* concentrated than 0.9% saline. These solutions are called "hypotonic". When hypotonic solutions are infused into the body, water *outside* the cell will flow toward the highest salt concentration (which is *inside* the cell). This forces water into dehydrated cells (see the picture below). The following list identifies the commercially available formulations of saline solutions.

   a. **Normal Saline (NS) – 0.9% Saline.** This *isotonic* solution contains 0.9 grams of sodium chloride (salt) per 100 mls of solution. This equivalent can be written as a fraction: 0.9 grams/100 mls.

   b. **½ NS (aka "half normal") – 0.45% Saline.** This *hypotonic* solution contains 0.45 grams of sodium chloride per 100 mls of solution (0.45 grams/100 mls). Since this solution contains a *lesser* concentration of salt than the normal body tissues, it forces water across the cell membranes and into the cells.

   c. **¼ NS (aka "quarter normal") – 0.225% Saline.** This *hypotonic* solution contains 0.225 grams of sodium chloride per 100 mls of solution (0.225 grams/100 mls). This solution also contains a *lesser* concentration of salt than normal body tissues, so water is forced into the cells.

Isotonic Solution   **Hypotonic Solution**

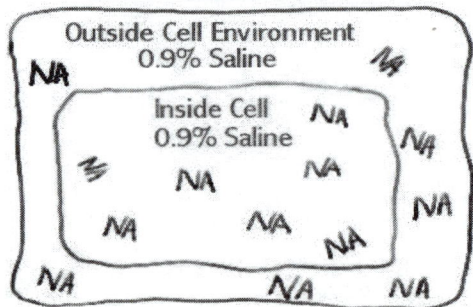
Because the sodium (NA) concentration is the same inside and outside the cell the water levels will remain the same inside and outside the cell.

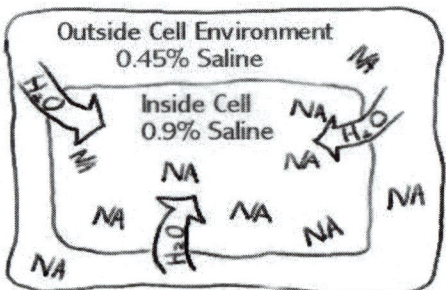
Because the sodium (NA) concentration inside the cell is greater than the concentration outside the cell, the water infuses into the cell. Remember: water follows salt!

3. **Lactated Ringers** (aka Ringer's Lactate, LR, RL) – This is a solution that contains sodium chloride, like a saline solution, but also small concentrations of potassium and calcium salts. Lactated Ringers are used to correct fluid and electrolyte imbalances/deficits. It is also common to see standard formulations of dextrose combined with lactated ringers. **Ex. D5LR (5% Dextrose in Lactated Ringers)**

4. **Sterile Water for Injection (SWFI)** – This is a water solution that has been sterilized and is pyrogen-free. SWFI contains no antimicrobial

agents or any other substances. This type of water is available in single-use containers of up to one-liter in size. This solution is intended for use as a diluent, solvent or vehicle for sterile injectable products. The one-liter bags *are not* intended for direct IV administration because they have no tonicity.

The above sterile solutions are packaged in both plastic IV bags and glass bottles. These bags and bottles are typically available from a manufacturer in sizes ranging from 50 mls to 3000 mls. They can also be found in many different combinations, like D5LR (5% Dextrose in Lactated Ringers) or D5NS (5% Dextrose in Normal Saline).

These solutions are very important by themselves, for fluid replacement, electrolyte balance restoration and supplemental nutrition. However, they also provide important vehicles for the administration of injectable drugs and total parenteral nutrition (TPN) admixtures, into the body.

Medications cannot be injected into just *any* bag of sterile IV fluid. Certain drugs are *not* compatible with certain IV solutions. In fact, some injectable drugs will "precipitate out" when introduced into a non-compatible IV solution. This means that the drug can form crystals or clumps at the bottom of the IV bag. Precipitate matter must never be introduced into a patient's vein. Therefore, it is of the utmost importance that the correct IV solution is chosen based on its compatibility with the injectable drug to be administered. An example of an incompatibility exists between injectable ampicillin and D5W (5% Dextrose in Water). This drug and this IV solution are *not* compatible. Ampicillin *must* be added to a bag of saline because it is not compatible with dextrose solutions. Drug/drug and drug/solution IV compatibility information can be easily accessed using a reference book such as "The Handbook on Injectable Drugs", (Trissel, L. et al).

IV solutions come in standard sizes that range from 50 mL bags to 3000 mL bags. Here are the standard sizes:

50 mL	**3000 mL**
100 mL	**1000 mL**
150 mL	**500 mL**
250 mL	

Rx Success™ Complete Guide to Medical Math

IV Drip Rate Calculations

IV drugs are most often ordered in terms of mL/hr. This determines how many milliliters of fluid are delivered into the patient per hour.

IV tubing, however, is not used to deliver milliliters of fluid, per se. Rather, IV tubing can be set to deliver a certain number of *drops* per min (gtts/min). There are various types of IV tubing, but each set has a hollow plastic chamber called a drip chamber. By looking at the drip chamber and counting, one can easily determine how many drops per minute the patient is receiving. The drops per minute can be adjusted manually or by machine.

Though it is important to know how many drops are being given to the patient per minute, it is just as important to know how *big* the drop is. IV tubing is calibrated in terms of drops per ml (gtts/ml). Or, how many drops it takes to equal 1 ml of fluid. This value is called the **drop factor**. The drop size depends on the size of the hole in the tubing. For instance: If the drop factor for Tubing A is marked 20 gtts/ml and the drop factor for Tubing B is marked 15 drops/ml, Tubing A's drops would be smaller than Tubing B's drops.

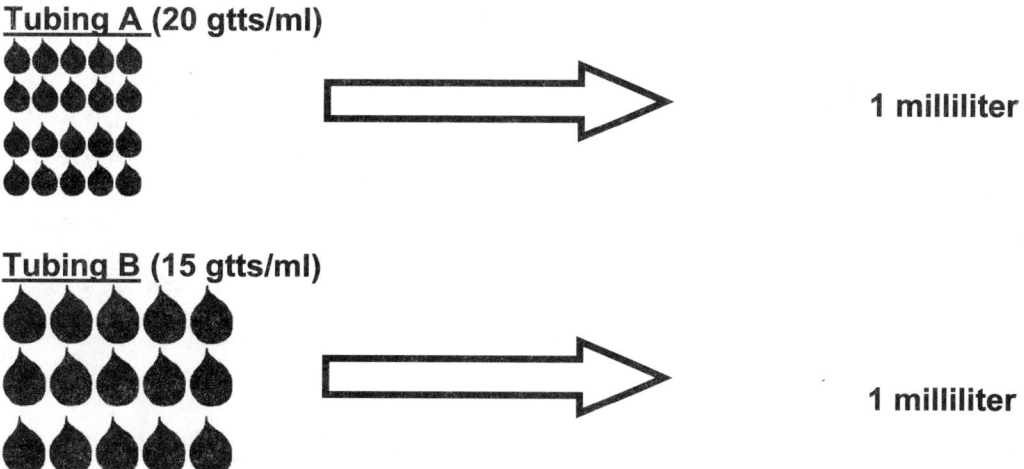

There is also IV tubing that is calibrated to deliver very tiny drops, called "microdrops". When this "microdrip" tubing is encountered, a drop factor of 60 gtts/ml must be used.

Perhaps the most important thing to remember when doing these calculations is to <u>always</u> keep in mind what units your answer needs to be in. If the problem asks for gtts/min, ml/hr or ml/min, keep this in mind at every step to make sure you are heading toward the correct answer.

IV drip rate calculations can generally be done in three (or fewer) steps, depending on where the problem begins. The steps are as follows:

Rx Success™ Complete Guide to Medical Math

- **STEP ONE:** Find ml/hour. It must be determined how many mls of IV fluid the patient is receiving in one hour. Remember, the problem may give you this information, so the first step may not be necessary.

- **STEP TWO:** Find ml/min. You must calculate how many mls of fluid the patient is receiving in one minute. In other words, when one minute has gone by, how many mls of fluid did the patient get? You will need to take the answer you got for step one (which is ml/hour) and change the "hour" on the bottom of the fraction into minutes. Since we know that one hour equals 60 minutes, the fraction becomes ml/60 min. We can then determine the number of mls per one minute using cross multiplication.

- **STEP THREE:** Find gtts/min (drops/min). It is very important to remember that you CANNOT move from **step two** to **step three** without one vital piece of information – the drop factor (based on the tubing being used for the administration of the IV). When performing the calculation on step three to find gtts/1 min, you will <u>always</u> use the drop factor as your "code" for the problem. The drop factor units will be in drops/ml. Some common drop factors are: 10 gtts/ml, 15 gtts/ml, 20 gtts/ml, 60 gtts/ml. The problem must provide this information if you are to calculate gtts/min. **Round all drops to the nearest whole number.**

<u>Don't be fooled!</u> Just because a problem provides you with a drop factor does not mean you will automatically complete all three steps! The problem may be looking for a final answer in ml/hr or ml/min (in which case, stop after step one or step two, respectively).

Calculating Total Infusion Time

When given the rate for an IV solution, you may be asked to calculate how long the entire IV will take to infuse (i.e. total infusion time). This is a relatively simple calculation, yet requires practice to increase your comfort level with these types of problems.

To calculate total infusion time, you *must* find an equivalent (fraction) that involves a volume amount of solution per some amount of time. Suppose you receive the following order and you are to calculate the total infusion time for this IV solution.

Order: A patient is to receive 1200 ml of NS, running at 45 gtts/min using 15 gtts/ml tubing. Calculate the total infusion time for this IV solution.

The problem provides the equivalent we need (volume of solution per some amount of time) to solve this problem when it says that the IV is, "…running at 45 gtts/min".

Rx Success™ Complete Guide to Medical Math

$$\frac{\text{45 gtts}}{\text{1 min}} \quad \text{(volume of solution)} \atop \text{(amount of time)}$$

This information tells us that the patient is receiving 45 gtts of fluid every minute. First, we'll use the drop factor (15 gtts/ml) as the code to convert 45 gtts into mls. Looks like this…

$$\frac{\text{15 gtts}}{\text{1 ml}} = \frac{\text{45 gtts}}{\text{X ml}}$$

(Handwritten work shown:)
X mL / 45 gtts = 1 mL / 15 gtts
15X = 45
X = 3 mL

X min / 1200 mL = 1 min / 3 mL
3X = 1200
X = 400 min

This calculation tells us that 45 gtts of solution is equal 3 mls of fluid. This means that the patient is receiving 3 ml of solution every minute (3 ml/min). Now, use this fraction to determine how many minutes it will take to infuse the entire 1200 ml solution.

$$\frac{\text{3 ml}}{\text{1 min}} = \frac{\text{1200 ml}}{\text{X min}}$$

We find that it will take a total of **400 min** to infuse the entire bag of fluid.

Calculating Amount of Drug Per Time

This type of calculation is performed when the problem asks how many strength units (whether they are grams, mg, mcg, units or mEq) of drug the patient will receive per period of time. To calculate the amount of drug the patient is receiving per unit of time, you *must* find an equivalent (fraction) that involves an amount of drug per some amount of time. For example, suppose the order stated…

Order: A 375 ml bag of D5W contains 650 mg of vancomycin to be infused over 4 hours using 20 gtts/ml tubing. How many mg of vancomycin will the patient receive every minute?

The problem asks us to calculate **mg/min** for this particular IV. Remember, the problem *must* provide, *or* you must calculate, an equivalent that involves a strength amount of drug per some amount of time. This problem provides that information when they tell us, "650 mg…to be infused over 4 hours". To write this as a "code", simply put this information in fraction form…

$$\frac{\text{650 mg}}{\text{4 hrs}} \quad \text{(amount of drug)} \atop \text{(amount of time)}$$

This fraction makes it very easy to calculate mg/min. First, we will convert 4 hours into 240 minutes. Now the fraction looks like this…

Rx Success™ Complete Guide to Medical Math

$$\frac{650 \text{ mg}}{240 \text{ min}}$$

And then, fill in the rest of the cross multiplication problem...

$$\frac{650 \text{ mg}}{240 \text{ min}} = \frac{X \text{ mg}}{1 \text{ min}}$$

And solve to get: **2.71 mg/min**

It is also important to see the extraneous information given in this problem that was not necessary to perform the calculation (i.e. the drop factor and the total number of mls in the IV solution). This information is not given simply to *trick* you. Were you to receive this as an actual order at work, you would need all of this information to provide the correct IV solution to the patient and to run it at the correct rate. Yet, to perform a necessary *calculation* with this information, you may not need everything given.

Remember...

To Calculate	*You Must Find...*
Total Infusion Time	**Volume of Solution/Time**
	Ex: 100 ml/hr
	Ex: 30 gtts/min
	Ex: 750 ml/6 hr
Amount of Drug per Time	**Amount of Drug/Time**
	Ex: 0.5 mg/min
	Ex: 5000 u/hr
	Ex: 40 mEq/4 hr

Study the Sample Problems in the pages that follow and complete the Tutor Sheets™. Then, you should be ready to complete the IV Drip Rate Calculations Homework at the end of this chapter.

Rx Success™ Complete Guide to Medical Math
IV Drip Rate Calculations - Sample Problems

1. Order: 1000 ml of D5W over 24 hrs. _____ ml/hr

   Using cross multiplication, 1000 ml per 24 hrs is the conversion factor to find how many ml per 1 hr.

   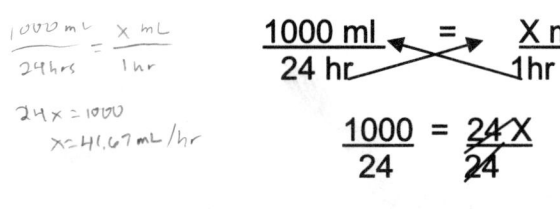

   $$\frac{1000 \text{ ml}}{24 \text{ hr}} = \frac{X \text{ ml}}{1 \text{ hr}}$$

   $$\frac{1000}{24} = \frac{24X}{24}$$

   X = 41.67

   Answer: 41.67 ml/hr

---

2. Order 500 ml Normal Saline to be infused over 16 hr. _____ ml/hr

   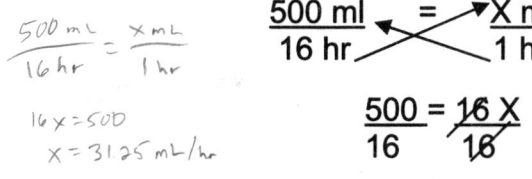

   $$\frac{500 \text{ ml}}{16 \text{ hr}} = \frac{X \text{ ml}}{1 \text{ hr}}$$

   $$\frac{500}{16} = \frac{16 X}{16}$$

   X = 31.25

   Answer: 31.25 ml/hr

---

3. Order: 1000 ml NS to be infused over 12 hrs. _____ ml/min

   This time the answer must be in ml/min rather than ml/hr. The first step is the same as the previous problems.

   $$\frac{X \text{ mL}}{1 \text{ min}} = \frac{1000 \text{ mL}}{720 \text{ min}}$$

   $720 X = 1000$

   $X = 1.39 \text{ mL/min}$

   $$\frac{1000 \text{ ml}}{12 \text{ hr}} = \frac{X \text{ ml}}{1 \text{ hr}}$$

   $$\frac{X \text{ mL}}{1 \text{ min}} = \frac{1000 \text{ mL}}{720 \text{ min}}$$

   $720 X = 1000$

   $X = 1.39 \text{ mL/min}$

   $$\frac{1000}{12} = \frac{12 X}{12}$$

   X = 83.3

Rx Success™ Complete Guide to Medical Math

The IV is running at 83.3 ml/hr. Now calculate ml/min. First, change 1 hr to 60 minutes. Then find ml per 1 min.

$$\frac{83.3 \text{ ml}}{60 \text{ min}} = \frac{X \text{ ml}}{1 \text{ min}}$$

$$\frac{83}{60} = \frac{60 X}{60}$$

X = 1.4

Answer: 1.4 ml/min

---

4. Order: 1500 ml to be infused over 4 hours. _____ml/min

$$\frac{1500 \text{ ml}}{4 \text{ hr}} = \frac{X \text{ ml}}{1 \text{ hr}}$$

$$\frac{1500}{4} = \frac{4X}{4}$$

X = 375 ml

Handwritten: $\frac{x\,mL}{1\,min} = \frac{1500\,mL}{240\,min}$; $240X = 1500$; $X = 6.25\,mL/min$

The IV is running at 375 ml/hr. Now find ml/min.

$$\frac{375 \text{ ml}}{60 \text{ min}} = \frac{X \text{ ml}}{1 \text{ min}}$$

$$\frac{375}{60} = \frac{60 X}{60}$$

X = 6.25

Handwritten: $\frac{x\,mL}{1\,min} = \frac{1500\,mL}{240\,min}$; $240x = 1500$; $X = 6.25\,mL/min$

Answer: 6.25 ml/min

---

5. Order: 1000 ml to be infused over 6 hrs. Use microdrip tubing.

Handwritten: $\frac{x\,mL}{1\,min} = \frac{1000\,mL}{360\,min}$; $360x = 1000$; $x = 2.78\,mL/min$; $\frac{x\,gtt}{2.78\,mL} = \frac{60\,gtt}{mL}$; $x = 167\,gtts/min$

_____gtts/min

The first two steps to the problem are the same as the previous problems. Here is the path to take.

Convert to: **ml/hr**   then   **ml/min**   then   **gtts/min**

Rx Success™ Complete Guide to Medical Math

a) $\dfrac{1000 \text{ ml}}{6 \text{ hr}} = \dfrac{X \text{ ml}}{1 \text{ hr}}$

$\dfrac{1000 \text{ ml}}{6} = \dfrac{\cancel{6}X}{\cancel{6}}$

X = 166.67   answer: 166.67 ml/hr

$\dfrac{X \text{ mL}}{1 \text{ min}} = \dfrac{1000 \text{ mL}}{360 \text{ min}}$

$360X = 1000$

$X = 2.78 \text{ mL/min}$

$\dfrac{X \text{ gtts}}{2.78 \text{ mL}} = \dfrac{60 \text{ gtt}}{1 \text{ mL}}$

$X = 166.8 \text{ gtts/min}$
or
167 gtts/min

b) $\dfrac{166.67 \text{ ml}}{60 \text{ min}} = \dfrac{X \text{ ml}}{1 \text{ min}}$

$\dfrac{167}{60} = \dfrac{\cancel{60}X}{\cancel{60}}$

X = 2.78   answer: 2.78 ml/min

c) Since you know how many ml the patient is receiving per minute, you just need to convert 3 mls into drops. The problem said that a microdrip tubing set is being used which means the drop factor is 60 gtts/ml.

$\dfrac{60 \text{ gtts}}{1 \text{ ml}} = \dfrac{X \text{ gtts}}{2.78 \text{ ml}}$

X = 167 gtts

So, 2.78 ml = 167 gtts.

Answer: The IV should be set to run at 167 gtts/min.

---

6. Order: 1500 ml to be infused over 12 hours, using 20 drop/ml tubing. _____ gtts/min

a) $\dfrac{1500 \text{ ml}}{12 \text{ hr}} = \dfrac{X \text{ ml}}{1 \text{ hr}}$

$\dfrac{X \text{ mL}}{1 \text{ hr}} = \dfrac{1500 \text{ mL}}{12 \text{ hr}}$

$12X = 1500$

$X = 125 \text{ mL/hr}$

$\dfrac{125 \text{ mL}}{60 \text{ min}} = \dfrac{X \text{ mL}}{\text{min}}$

$60X = 125$

$X = 2.08 \text{ mL/min}$

$\dfrac{X \text{ gtt}}{2.08 \text{ mL}} = \dfrac{20 \text{ gtt}}{1 \text{ mL}}$

$X = 42 \text{ gtts/min}$

$\dfrac{X \text{ mL}}{1 \text{ min}} = \dfrac{1500 \text{ mL}}{720 \text{ min}}$

$720X = 1500$

$X = 2.08 \text{ mL/min}$

$\dfrac{X \text{ gtt}}{2.08 \text{ mL}} = \dfrac{20 \text{ gtt}}{1 \text{ mL}}$

$X = 41.6 \text{ gtt/min}$
or
42 gtt/min

Rx Success™ Complete Guide to Medical Math

$$\frac{1500}{12} = \frac{12X}{12}$$

X = 125   answer: 125 ml/hr

b) $\frac{125 \text{ ml}}{60 \text{ min}} = \frac{X \text{ ml}}{1 \text{ min}}$

$$\frac{125}{60} = \frac{60X}{60}$$

X = 2.08   answer: 2.08 ml/min

c) How many drops are in 2.08 ml?

$\frac{20 \text{ gtts}}{1 \text{ ml}} = \frac{X \text{ gtts}}{2.08 \text{ ml}}$

X = 41.6 gtts

Answer: The IV should be set at 42 gtts/min.

---

7. A 1250 ml IV contains 1000 mg of dobutamine and is running at 120 gtts/min. The nurse is using 20 gtts/ml tubing. Calculate the total infusion time for this IV.

    a) First, convert 120 gtts into mls. This will determine the infusion rate in ml/min. Use the drop factor (20 gtts/ml) as the code.

    $$\frac{20 \text{ gtts}}{1 \text{ ml}} = \frac{120 \text{ gtts}}{X \text{ ml}}$$

    Once completed, you find that 120 gtts = 6 ml. This means that the patient is receiving 6 ml/min.

Rx Success™ Complete Guide to Medical Math

b) Finally, use the drip rate found in the first step (6 ml/min) as the code to calculate the total infusion time.

$$\frac{6 \text{ ml}}{1 \text{ min}} = \frac{1250 \text{ ml}}{X \text{ min}}$$

When this calculation is finished, we find that the total infusion time is **208.3 min**.

---

8. A patient is to receive 800 ml of D5W containing 1200 mg of dopamine to be infused over 8 hours. How many mg of dopamine will the patient receive per minute?

   a) First, notice that the problem tells us that 1200 mg of dopamine is to be infused over 8 hours. In this particular problem, we are only concerned with the amount of "drug" in the bag, *not* the fluid volume. Write this as a fraction (1200 mg/8 hrs) and use it as a code to determine how many mg the patient is receiving per one hour.

   [handwritten margin work:]
   $\frac{1200 \text{ mg}}{8 \text{ hr}} = \frac{X \text{ mg}}{1 \text{ hr}}$
   $8x = 1200$
   $x = 150 \text{ mg/hr}$

   $$\frac{1200 \text{ mg}}{8 \text{ hr}} = \frac{X \text{ mg}}{1 \text{ hr}}$$

   [handwritten right margin:]
   $\frac{X \text{ mg}}{1 \text{ min}} = \frac{1200 \text{ mg}}{480 \text{ min}}$
   $480x = 1200$
   $x = 2.5 \text{ mg/min}$

   [handwritten lower left:]
   $\frac{X \text{ mg}}{1 \text{ min}} = \frac{150 \text{ mg}}{60 \text{ min}}$
   $60x = 150$
   $x = 2.5 \text{ mg/min}$

   Once completed, you find that the patient is receiving 150 mg per hour (150 mg/1 hr).

   b) Now, convert the "1 hr" to "60 min" in the fraction you found for the first step. The fraction now looks like this: 150 mg/60 min. Use this new fraction as the code to calculate mg/min.

   $$\frac{150 \text{ mg}}{60 \text{ min}} = \frac{X \text{ mg}}{1 \text{ min}}$$

   Once completed, you find that the patient is receiving 2.5 mg per minute **(2.5 mg/min)**.

---

9. A solution of heparin 25,000 units in D5W 500 mL is running at 25 ml/hr. How many units of heparin will the patient receive every hour?

   For this and other IV calculations, it can be extremely helpful to draw the IV bag and label it. The bag will generally have *two* components: the amount of drug and the amount of fluid. In this case, the IV bag is labeled like this:

   [handwritten margin work:]
   $\frac{XU}{25 \text{ mL}} = \frac{25000 U}{500 \text{ mL}}$
   $500x = 625000$
   $x = 1250 \text{ U/hr}$

   $\frac{XU}{25 \text{ mL}} = \frac{25000}{500 \text{ mL}}$
   $500x = 625000$
   $x = 1250 \text{ U/hr}$

Rx Success™ Complete Guide to Medical Math

25,000 U/500 ml. Now, look at the information that the problem provides and what you are being asked to find. The problem says that the IV is running at 25 ml/hr and we have to convert that to "units/hr". To complete this, the only step that needs to be done is to convert 25 ml into units. This can be done easily by using the "code" that is on our drawing of the IV bag (25,000 U/500 ml).

$$\frac{25{,}000 \text{ U}}{500 \text{ ml}} = \frac{X \text{ U}}{25 \text{ ml}}$$

After completing this problem, we know that 25 ml is equal to 1250 U of heparin. So we simply replace the 25 ml with 1250 U and our final answer is: **1250 U/hr**.

---

10. A 46 lb patient requires aminophylline IV at a rate of 1.2 mg/kg/hr. The IV solution contains 400 mg of aminophylline in 500 ml of D5W. Determine the correct IV flow rate in ml/hr.

    a) Take notice when the order says that every hour, the pt needs to receive 1.2 mg/1 kg of drug. Next, draw the IV bag and label it properly with both components (400 mg/500 ml).

    b) Now, we must calculate how many mg of drug the patient is going to receive per hour, based on the patient's weight. The order says per **kg** of body weight yet the patient's weight is provided in lbs. This requires us to convert the patient's weight to kg before we can determine how much drug they need per hour.

$$\frac{2.2 \text{ lb}}{1 \text{ kg}} = \frac{46 \text{ lb}}{X \text{ kg}}$$

    After the calculation, we find that the patient weighs **20.91** kg.

    c) Now, take the order (1.2 mg/kg) and the patient weight in kg and determine how many mg of drug they must receive each hour.

$$\frac{1.2 \text{ mg}}{1 \text{ kg}} = \frac{X \text{ mg}}{20.91 \text{ kg}}$$

    After the calculation, we find that the patient requires 25.09 mg of drug, per hour (25.09 mg/1 hr).

Rx Success™ Complete Guide to Medical Math

d) Now, we must convert the 25.09 mg into mls. To perform this calculation, we must find a fraction (code) that provides an equivalent between mg and mls. Look back at the IV bag that you have drawn. It should be labeled with: 400 mg/500 mls. This is the code we will use.

$$\frac{400 \text{ mg}}{500 \text{ ml}} = \frac{25.09 \text{ mg}}{X \text{ ml}}$$

And we find that 25.09 mg is equal to **31.36 ml**. Finally, we simply replace the 25.09 mg with 31.36 ml and the final fraction becomes **31.36 ml/1 hr**.

$$\frac{X \text{ ml}}{25.09 \text{ mg}} = \frac{500 \text{ mL}}{400 \text{ mg}}$$

400X = 12545
X = 31.36 mL/hr

$$\frac{X \text{ kg}}{46 \text{ lb}} = \frac{1 \text{ kg}}{2.2 \text{ lb}}$$

2.2X = 46
X = 20.91 kg

$$\frac{X \text{ mg}}{20.91 \text{ kg}} = \frac{1.2 \text{ mg}}{1 \text{ kg}}$$

X = 25.09 mg/hr

$$\frac{X \text{ mL}}{25.09 \text{ mg}} = \frac{500 \text{ mL}}{400 \text{ mg}}$$

400X = 12545
X = 31.36 mL/hr

Rx Success™ Complete Guide to Medical Math

IV Drip Rate Calculations – Tutor Sheets™

USE THIS WORKSHEET AS A GUIDE TO HELP YOU SOLVE THE HOMEWORK PROBLEMS!

1. Order: 350 mL of D5W over 4 hrs. Calculate the flow rate in ml/hr.

    Write a fraction from the information given in the problem and use it as the code for a cross multiplication problem to calculation the flow rate in ml/hr.

    $\dfrac{X\ mL}{1\ hr} = \dfrac{350\ mL}{4\ hr}$

    $4x = 350$

    $x = 87.5\ mL/hr$

    $\dfrac{ml}{hr} \times \dfrac{X\ ml}{1\ hr}$

    _____ = _____

    $\dfrac{X\ mL}{1\ hr} = \dfrac{350\ mL}{4\ hr}$

    $4x = 350$

    $x = 87.5\ mL/hr$

    = _____ ml/hr

---

2. Order: 1.8 L of NS to be infused over 10 hr. Calculate the flow rate in ml/min.

    Step One – Notice that the problem requires the flow rate to be calculated in **ml** per min. Yet, the fluid volume of the solution, in the problem, is in **Liters**. Therefore, prior to the first step, we must first convert the volume of solution into ml.

    $\dfrac{X\ mL}{1\ min} = \dfrac{1800\ mL}{600\ min}$

    1.8 L = _____ ml

    $600x = 1800$

    $x = 3\ mL/min$

    Now, create a fraction from the information given in the problem (do not forget to list the fluid volume in ml, *not* Liters). Use this fraction as the code for a cross multiplication problem to calculate ml/hr.

    $\dfrac{ml}{hr} \times \dfrac{X\ ml}{1\ hr}$

    _____ = _____

    $\dfrac{X\ mL}{1\ min} = \dfrac{1800\ mL}{600\ min}$

    $600x = 1800$

    $x = 3\ mL/min$

    = _____ ml/hr

Page - 205

Rx Success™ Complete Guide to Medical Math

Step Two – Step one gave us a fraction in "ml/hr". Convert the bottom of the fraction into minutes by replacing "1 hr" with "60 min". Then, use that fraction as a code for a cross multiplication problem to calculate ml/min.

$$\frac{\text{ml}}{60 \text{ min}} = \frac{X \text{ ml}}{1 \text{ min}}$$

_____ = _____

= _____ ml/min

---

3. A patient is to receive 275 ml of 5% Dextrose in Water with 200 mg of ciprofloxacin over 3 hours using IV tubing calibrated to deliver 15 gtts/ml. Calculate the flow rate in gtts/min.

    Step One – Set up a cross multiplication problem with information from the problem to calculate ml/1 hr.

$$\frac{X\,mL}{1\,min} = \frac{275\,mL}{180\,min}$$

$$180x = 275$$

$$x = 1.53\,mL/min$$

$$\frac{X\,gtt}{1.53\,mL} = \frac{15\,gtt}{1\,mL}$$

$$x = 22.95\,gtt/min$$

or 23 gtt/min

$$\frac{\text{ml}}{\text{hr}} = \frac{X \text{ ml}}{1 \text{ hr}}$$

$$\frac{X\,mL}{1\,min} = \frac{275\,mL}{180\,min}$$

$$180x = 275$$

$$x = 1.53\,mL/min$$

$$\frac{X\,gtt}{1.53\,mL} = \frac{15\,gtt}{1\,mL} \quad x = 22.95\,gtt/min$$

or 23 gtt/min

_____ = _____ ml/hr

Step Two – Convert 1 hr to 60 minutes and set up a second cross multiplication problem to calculate ml/1 min

$$\frac{\text{ml}}{60 \text{ min}} = \frac{X \text{ ml}}{1 \text{ min}}$$

Rx Success™ Complete Guide to Medical Math

_____ = _____

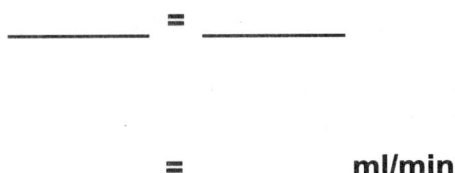

= _____ ml/min

Step Three – Identify the drop factor from the problem. Use the drop factor as the code for the next cross multiplication problem to convert the number of **ml** per min (found in step 2) to **drops** per minute.

$$\frac{\text{gtts}}{1 \text{ ml}} = \frac{X \text{ gtts}}{\text{ml}}$$

_____ = _____

= _____ gtts

Now, replace the number of mls in the fraction you found for step 2, with the number of drops you found in step 3.

= _____ gtts/min

---

4. An 1100 ml bag of IV fluid that contains 40 mEq of KCl is running at 90 gtts/min through IV tubing calibrated to deliver 20 gtts/ml. Calculate the total infusion time for this IV.

Step One – The problem tells us that the IV is currently running at 90 gtts/ml. Use the drop factor given in the problem to convert 90 gtts into ml. This will tell you how many ml of fluid the patient is receiving every minute.

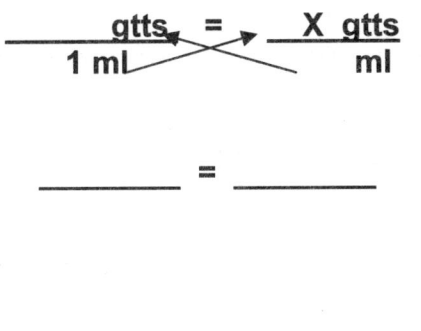

$$\frac{\text{gtts}}{1 \text{ ml}} = \frac{90 \text{ gtts}}{X \text{ ml}}$$

$\frac{X \text{ min}}{1100 \text{ mL}} = \frac{1 \text{ min}}{4.5 \text{ mL}}$ $4.5x = 1100$

$X = 244.44 \text{ min}$

$\frac{X \text{ mL}}{90 \text{ gtt}} = \frac{1 \text{ mL}}{20 \text{ gtt}}$ $20x = 90$

$X = 4.5 \text{ mL/min}$

$\frac{X \text{ min}}{1100 \text{ mL}} = \frac{1 \text{ min}}{4.5 \text{ mL}}$ $4.5x = 1100$

$X = 244.44 \text{ mins}$

Rx Success™ Complete Guide to Medical Math

_____ = _____

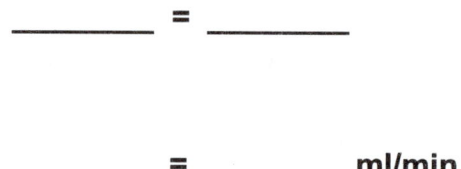

= _____ ml/min

Step Two – Take the fraction found in step one and use it as the code for a cross multiplication problem that will tell you how many minutes it will take to infuse the entire 1100 ml of fluid.

$$\frac{\text{ml}}{\text{min}} \bowtie \frac{1100 \text{ ml}}{X \text{ min}}$$

_____ = _____

= _____ min

---

5. A 250 ml bag of D5W contains 1 g of lidocaine to be infused over 8 hours using 20 gtts/ml tubing. Calculate how many mg of lidocaine the patient will receive every minute.

$\frac{X \text{ mg}}{1 \text{ min}} = \frac{1000 \text{ mg}}{480 \text{ min}}$

$480X = 1000$

$x = 2.08 \text{ mg/min}$

Step One – Notice that the problem requires the amount of drug to be calculated in **mg** per min. Yet, the strength amount of the drug in the problem, is given in **grams**. Therefore, prior to the first step, we must first convert the amount of drug in solution to mg.

$$1 \text{ g} = \underline{\quad 1000 \quad} \text{ mg}$$

Now, create a fraction from the information given in the problem (do not forget to list the amount of drug in mg, *not* grams). Use this fraction as the code for a cross multiplication problem to calculate the number of mg/hr the patient is receiving.

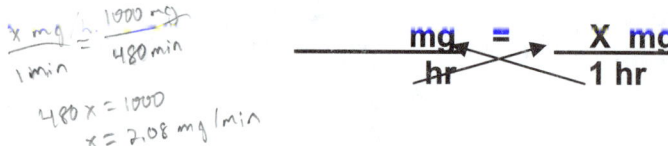

$\frac{\text{mg}}{\text{hr}} \bowtie \frac{X \text{ mg}}{1 \text{ hr}}$

$\frac{X \text{ mg}}{1 \text{ min}} = \frac{1000 \text{ mg}}{480 \text{ min}}$

$480X = 1000$

$x = 2.08 \text{ mg/min}$

Rx Success™ Complete Guide to Medical Math

$$\underline{\qquad} = \underline{\qquad}$$

$$= \underline{\qquad} \text{mg/hr}$$

Step Two – Step one gave us a fraction in "mg/hr". Convert the bottom of the fraction into minutes by replacing "1 hr" with "60 min". Then, use that fraction as a code for a cross multiplication problem to calculate the number of mg/min.

$$\frac{mg}{60\ min} ⤫ \frac{X\ mg}{1\ min}$$

$$\underline{\qquad} = \underline{\qquad}$$

$$= \underline{\qquad} \text{mg/min}$$

---

6. A patient is to receive 125 mg of nitroglycerin in 500 ml of D5W at a rate of 42 mcg/min. Calculate the flow rate in ml/hr.

   Step One – Draw and label the IV bag with the amount of fluid *and* the amount of drug. Notice that the amount of drug in the IV bag is in **mg** but the amount of drug the patient receives per min (42 mcg/min) is in **mcg**. Therefore, we must first convert *either* the amount of drug in the IV bag to mcg, *or* convert the 42 mcg into mg. So long as the two units match, it does not matter which you convert. For this problem, we are going to convert 42 mcg to mg.

   42 mcg = __0.042__ mg

   Now, create a fraction from the information you just found, telling you how many mg the patient receives per min.

   $$\frac{\underline{\qquad}\ mg}{min}$$

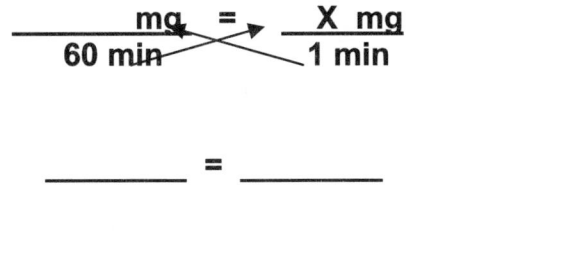

Rx Success™ Complete Guide to Medical Math

Step Two – Now, you must convert the number of mg the patient receives per minute into ml. To perform this calculation we must have a code between ml and mg. This code should be on the IV bag that you have drawn and labeled.

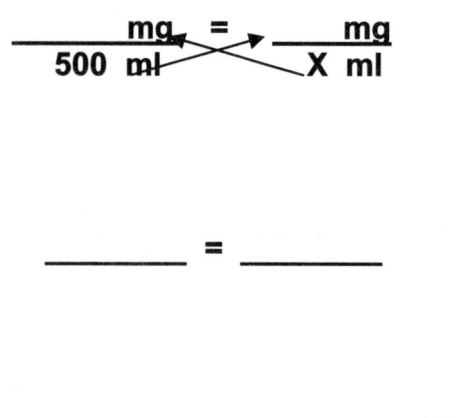

_____ = _____

= _____ ml/hr

Answers to Tutor Sheets™ Calculations
1) 87.5 ml/hr   2) 3 ml/min   3) 23 gtts/min   4) 244.44 min   5) 2.08 mg/min   6) 10.2 ml/hr

Rx Success™ Complete Guide to Medical Math

IV Drip Rate Calculations - Homework

Calculate the following IV drip rates. Be careful to note the units.

1. A 600 ml IV is scheduled to run over 4 hours. Calculate the flow rate in ml/hr.

   $$\frac{x\ ml}{1\ hr} = \frac{600\ mL}{4\ hr} \qquad 4x = 600 \qquad x = 150\ ml/hr$$

   _____150_____ ml/hr

2. A 1250 ml bag of 20% Dextrose solution is to be infused over 5 hours. Calculate the flow rate in ml/hr.

   $$\frac{x\ mL}{1\ hr} = \frac{1250\ mL}{5\ hr} \qquad 5x = 1250 \qquad x = 250\ mL/hr$$

   _____250_____ ml/hr

3. A 150 ml bag of D5W is to be infused over 2 hours, using 15 gtts/ml tubing. Calculate the flow rate in ml/min.

   $$\frac{x\ mL}{1\ hr} = \frac{150\ mL}{2\ hr} \qquad 2x = 150 \qquad x = 75\ mL/hr$$

   $$\frac{x\ mL}{min} = \frac{75\ mL}{60\ min} \qquad 60x = 75 \qquad x = 1.25\ mL/min$$

   _____1.25_____ ml/min

4. A patient is to receive 800 ml of 0.9% Saline over 4 hours using IV tubing calibrated to 10 gtts/ml. Calculate the flow rate in ml/min and gtts/min.

   $$\frac{x\ mL}{1\ min} = \frac{800\ mL}{240\ min} \qquad 240x = 800 \qquad x = 3.33\ mL/min$$

   $$\frac{x\ gtt}{3.33\ mL} = \frac{10\ gtt}{1\ mL} \qquad x = 33\ gtts/min$$

   _____3.33_____ ml/min

   _____33_____ gtts/min

5. A 100 ml antibiotic piggyback is to be infused over 1 hour using microdrip tubing. Calculate the flow rate in ml/min and gtts/min.

   $$\frac{x\ mL}{1\ min} = \frac{100\ mL}{60\ min} \qquad 60x = 100 \qquad x = 1.67\ mL/min$$

   $$\frac{x\ gtt}{1.67\ mL} = \frac{60\ gtt}{1\ mL} \qquad x = 100\ gtts/min$$

   _____1.67_____ ml/min

   _____100_____ gtts/min

Rx Success™ Complete Guide to Medical Math

6. Calculate the flow rate in gtts/min for a 1000 ml bag of 5% amino acid solution that is to be infused over 6 hours, using 20 gtts/ml tubing.

$$\frac{X\ mL}{1\ min} = \frac{1000\ mL}{360\ min} \qquad 360X = 1000$$
$$X = 2.78\ mL/min$$

$$\frac{X\ gtt}{2.78\ mL} = \frac{20\ gtt}{1\ mL} \qquad X = 56\ gtts/min$$

__56__ gtts/min

7. A patient is to receive 1000 mg of dobutamine in 500 ml of D5W over 2 hours using 12 gtts/ml tubing. Calculate the flow rate in ml/min and gtts/min.

$$\frac{X\ mL}{1\ min} = \frac{500\ mL}{120\ min} \qquad 120X = 500$$
$$X = 4.17\ mL/min$$

$$\frac{X\ gtt}{4.17\ mL} = \frac{12\ gtt}{mL} \qquad X = 50\ gtts/min$$

__4.17__ ml/min

__50__ gtts/min

8. A patient is to receive 750 mg of ciprofloxacin in 150 ml of NS. The IV is to run over 3 hours using 30 gtts/ml tubing. Calculate the flow rate in ml/min and gtts/min.

$$\frac{X\ mL}{1\ min} = \frac{150\ mL}{180\ min} \qquad 180X = 150$$
$$X = 0.83\ mL/min$$

$$\frac{X\ gtt}{0.83\ mL} = \frac{30\ gtt}{1\ mL} \qquad X = 25\ gtts/min$$

__0.83__ ml/min

__25__ gtts/min

9. A 250 ml IV containing 500 mg of vancomycin is to be infused over three hours, using 10 gtts/ml tubing. Calculate the flow rate in ml/min.

$$\frac{X\ mL}{1\ min} = \frac{250\ mL}{180\ min} \qquad 180X = 250$$
$$X = 1.39\ mL/min$$

$$\frac{X\ gtt}{1.39\ mL} = \frac{10\ gtt}{1\ mL} \qquad X = 14\ gtts/min$$

__1.39__ ml/min

__14__ gtts/min

Rx Success™ Complete Guide to Medical Math

10. A patient is to receive 1200 ml of 0.9% saline over six hours using 15 gtts/ml tubing. Calculate the flow rate in ml/min and gtts/min.

$$\frac{X\,mL}{1\,min} = \frac{1200\,mL}{360\,min} \qquad 360x = 1200 \qquad x = 3.33\,mL/min$$

$$\frac{X\,gtt}{3.33\,mL} = \frac{15\,gtt}{1\,mL} \qquad x = 50\,gtts/min$$

_____3.33_____ ml/min

_____50_____ gtts/min

11. A 1 Liter bag of D5W is to be infused over four hours using IV tubing calibrated to 20 gtts/ml. Calculate the flow rate in ml/min and gtts/min.

$$\frac{X\,mL}{1\,min} = \frac{1000\,mL}{240\,min} \qquad 240x = 1000 \qquad x = 4.17\,mL/min$$

$$\frac{X\,gtt}{4.17\,mL} = \frac{20\,gtt}{1\,mL} \qquad x = 83\,gtts/min$$

_____4.17_____ ml/min

_____83_____ gtts/min

12. A 750 ml IV is to be infused over six hours using microdrip tubing. Calculate the flow rate in ml/min and gtts/min.

$$\frac{X\,mL}{1\,min} = \frac{750\,mL}{360\,min} \qquad 360x = 750 \qquad x = 2.08\,mL/min$$

$$\frac{X\,gtt}{2.08\,mL} = \frac{60\,gtt}{1\,mL} \qquad x = 125\,gtts/min$$

_____2.08_____ ml/min

_____125_____ gtts/min

13. A patient is to receive 1800 ml of fluid over 12 hours using IV tubing calibrated to 12 gtts/ml. Calculate the flow rate in ml/min and gtts/min.

$$\frac{X\,mL}{1\,min} = \frac{1800\,mL}{720\,min} \qquad 720x = 1800 \qquad x = 2.5\,mL/min$$

$$\frac{X\,gtt}{2.5\,mL} = \frac{12\,gtts}{1\,mL} \qquad x = 30\,gtts/min$$

_____2.5_____ ml/min

_____30_____ gtts/min

Rx Success™ Complete Guide to Medical Math

14. A 50 ml IVPB (IV piggyback) is to be infused over 30 minutes using 15 gtts/ml tubing. Calculate the flow rate in ml/min and gtts/min.

$$\frac{X\,mL}{1\,min} = \frac{50\,mL}{30\,min}$$

$30x = 50$

$x = 1.67\,mL/min$

$$\frac{X\,gtts}{1.67\,mL} = \frac{15\,gtt}{1\,mL}$$

$x = 25\,gtts/min$

_____1.67_____ ml/min

_____25_____ gtts/min

15. A 2.7 L TPN (total parenteral nutrition) is to run over 10 hours using 12 gtts/ml tubing. Calculate the flow rate in gtts/min.

$$\frac{X\,mL}{1\,min} = \frac{2700\,mL}{600\,min}$$

$600x = 2700$

$x = 4.5\,mL/min$

$$\frac{X\,gtt}{4.5\,mL} = \frac{12\,gtt}{1\,mL}$$

$x = 54\,gtts/min$

_____54_____ gtts/min

16. A patient is to receive 150 ml of NS over three hours using microdrip tubing. Calculate the flow rate in ml/min and gtts/min.

$$\frac{X\,mL}{1\,min} = \frac{150\,mL}{180\,min}$$

$180x = 150$

$x = 0.83\,mL/min$

$$\frac{X\,gtt}{0.83\,mL} = \frac{60\,gtt}{1\,mL}$$

$x = 50\,gtts/min$

_____0.83_____ ml/min

_____50_____ gtts/min

17. A 225 ml solution containing 800 mg of dopamine is to be infused over two hours using 15 gtts/ml tubing. Calculate the flow rate in ml/min and gtts/min.

$$\frac{X\,mL}{1\,min} = \frac{225\,mL}{120\,min}$$

$120x = 225$

$x = 1.88\,mL/min$

$$\frac{X\,gtt}{1.88\,mL} = \frac{15\,gtt}{1\,mL}$$

$x = 28.2\,gtts/min$

_____1.88_____ ml/min

_____28_____ gtts/min

Rx Success™ Complete Guide to Medical Math

18. A patient is to receive 45 U of Regular insulin in 150 ml of NS over five hours using tubing calibrated to deliver 10 gtts/ml. Calculate the flow rate in ml/min and gtts/min.

$$\frac{x\,mL}{1\,min} = \frac{150\,mL}{300\,min}$$
$$300x = 150$$
$$x = 0.5\,mL/min$$

$$\frac{x\,gtt}{0.5\,mL} = \frac{10\,gtt}{1\,mL}$$
$$x = 5\,gtt/min$$

_____0.5_____ ml/min

_____5_____ gtts/min

19. A patient is to receive 80 mEq of KCl (potassium chloride) in 1000 ml of 5% Dextrose in Water. The entire IV is to be infused over 5 hours using 10 gtts/ml tubing. Calculate the flow rate in ml/min and gtts/min.

$$\frac{x\,mL}{1\,min} = \frac{1000\,mL}{300\,min}$$
$$300x = 1000$$
$$x = 3.33\,mL/min$$

$$\frac{x\,gtt}{3.33\,mL} = \frac{10\,gtt}{1\,mL}$$
$$x = 33\,gtt/min$$

_____3.33_____ ml/min

_____33_____ gtts/min

20. A 500 ml bag of 0.9% Normal Saline, containing 25,000 units of heparin, is to be infused over 2 hours using microdrip tubing. Calculate the flow rate in ml/min and gtts/min.

$$\frac{x\,mL}{1\,min} = \frac{500\,mL}{120\,min}$$
$$120x = 500$$
$$x = 4.17\,mL/min$$

$$\frac{x\,gtt}{4.17\,mL} = \frac{60\,gtt}{1\,mL}$$
$$x = 250\,gtt/min$$

_____4.17_____ ml/min

_____250_____ gtts/min

Rx Success™ Complete Guide to Medical Math

Calculate the following total infusion times from the information given.

	Volume of IV	Rate	Drop Factor	Total Infusion Time
1.	350 ml	1.5 ml/min	not given	233.33 min
2.	1200 ml	8 ml/min	20 gtts/ml	150 min
3.	150 ml	5 ml/min	microdrip tubing	30 min
4.	225 ml	27 gtts/min	10 gtts/ml	83.33 min
5.	0.75 L	12 ml/min	not given	62.5 min
6.	0.25 L	120 gtts/min	30 gtts/ml	62.5 min
7.	3.4 L	90 gtts/min	15 gtts/ml	566.67 min
8.	2050 ml	64 gtts/min	12 gtts/ml	384.62 min
9.	1125 ml	45 gtts/min	20 gtts/ml	500 min
10.	0.48 L	112 gtts/min	15 gtts/ml	64.26 min

Rx Success™ Complete Guide to Medical Math

11. A 500 ml bag of D5W is running at 10 ml/min. Calculate the total infusion time.

    $\dfrac{x \text{ min}}{500 \text{ mL}} = \dfrac{1 \text{ min}}{10 \text{ mL}}$ $10x = 500$ $x = 50 \text{ min}$

    $\dfrac{x \text{ min}}{500 \text{ mL}} = \dfrac{1 \text{ min}}{10 \text{ mL}}$ $10x = 500$ $x = 50 \text{ min}$

    _____50_____ min

12. Calculate the total infusion time for a 1000 ml IV running at 7 ml/min.

    $\dfrac{x \text{ min}}{1000 \text{ mL}} = \dfrac{1 \text{ min}}{7 \text{ mL}}$ $7x = 1000$ $x = 142.86 \text{ min}$

    $\dfrac{x \text{ min}}{1000 \text{ mL}} = \dfrac{1 \text{ min}}{7 \text{ mL}}$ $7x = 1000$ $x = 142.86 \text{ min}$

    _____142.86_____ min

13. A 1.7 L TPN is running at 15 ml/min. Calculate the total infusion time.

    $\dfrac{x \text{ min}}{1700 \text{ mL}} = \dfrac{1 \text{ min}}{15 \text{ mL}}$ $15x = 1700$ $x = 113.33 \text{ min}$

    $\dfrac{x \text{ min}}{1700 \text{ mL}} = \dfrac{1 \text{ min}}{15 \text{ mL}}$

    $15x = 1700$

    $x = 113.33 \text{ min}$

    _____113.33_____ min

14. A 2.8 L bag of 0.45% Normal Saline is running at 180 gtts/min through IV tubing calibrated at 15 gtts/ml. Calculate the total infusion time.

    $\dfrac{x \text{ mL}}{180 \text{ gtt}} = \dfrac{1 \text{ mL}}{15 \text{ gtt}}$ $15x = 180$ $x = 12 \text{ mL/min}$

    $\dfrac{x \text{ min}}{2800 \text{ mL}} = \dfrac{1 \text{ min}}{12 \text{ mL}}$ $12x = 2800$ $x = 233.33 \text{ min}$

    $\dfrac{x \text{ mL}}{180 \text{ gtt}} = \dfrac{1 \text{ mL}}{15 \text{ gtt}}$ $15x = 180$ $x = 12 \text{ mL/min}$

    $\dfrac{x \text{ min}}{2800 \text{ mL}} = \dfrac{1 \text{ min}}{12 \text{ mL}}$ $12x = 2800$ $x = 233.33 \text{ min}$

    _____233.33_____ min

15. A 1250 ml IV contains 40 mEq of KCl and is running at 125 gtts/min through 30 gtts/ml tubing. Calculate the total infusion time for this IV.

    $\dfrac{x \text{ mL}}{125 \text{ gtt}} = \dfrac{1 \text{ mL}}{30 \text{ gtt}}$ $30x = 125$ $x = 4.17 \text{ mL/min}$

    $\dfrac{x \text{ min}}{1250 \text{ mL}} = \dfrac{1 \text{ min}}{4.17 \text{ mL}}$ $4.17x = 1250$ $x = 299.76 \text{ min}$

    $\dfrac{x \text{ mL}}{125 \text{ gtt}} = \dfrac{1 \text{ mL}}{30 \text{ gtt}}$ $30x = 125$ $x = 4.17 \text{ mL/min}$

    $\dfrac{x \text{ min}}{1250 \text{ mL}} = \dfrac{1 \text{ min}}{4.17 \text{ mL}}$ $4.17x = 1250$ $x = 299.76 \text{ min}$

    _____300_____ min

16. A 0.2 L bag of NS is running at 25 gtts/min using 15 gtts/ml tubing. Calculate the total infusion time for this IV.

    200 mL

    $\dfrac{x \text{ mL}}{25 \text{ gtt}} = \dfrac{1 \text{ mL}}{15 \text{ gtt}}$ $15x = 25$ $x = 1.67 \text{ mL/min}$

    $\dfrac{x \text{ min}}{200 \text{ mL}} = \dfrac{1 \text{ min}}{1.67 \text{ mL}}$ $1.67x = 200$ $x = 119.76 \text{ min}$

    $\dfrac{x \text{ mL}}{25 \text{ gtt}} = \dfrac{1 \text{ mL}}{15 \text{ gtt}}$ $\dfrac{x \text{ min}}{200 \text{ mL}} = \dfrac{1 \text{ min}}{1.67 \text{ mL}}$

    $15x = 25$ $1.67x = 200$

    $x = 1.67 \text{ mL/min}$ $x = 119.76 \text{ min}$

    _____120_____ min

Rx Success™ Complete Guide to Medical Math

17. A patient is to receive 500 mg of dobutamine in 500 ml of NS through 30 gtts/ml tubing. The IV is currently running at 75 gtts/min. Calculate the total infusion time for the entire bag of fluid.

$$\frac{X\,mL}{75\,gtt} = \frac{1\,mL}{30\,gtt} \qquad 30x = 75$$
$$x = 2.5\,mL/min$$

$$\frac{X\,min}{500\,mL} = \frac{1\,min}{2.5\,mL} \qquad 2.5x = 500$$
$$x = 200\,min$$

__200__ min

18. A patient is to receive 25,000 U of heparin in 700 ml of D5W. The IV is currently running at 90 gtts/min through 10 gtts/ml tubing. Calculate the total infusion time.

$$\frac{X\,mL}{90\,gtt} = \frac{1\,mL}{10\,gtt} \qquad 10x = 90$$
$$x = 9\,mL/min$$

$$\frac{X\,min}{700\,mL} = \frac{1\,min}{9\,mL} \qquad 9x = 700$$
$$x = 77.78\,min$$

__77.78__ min

19. A patient is receiving a 600 ml IV running at 105 gtts/min. Calculate the total infusion time if the tubing is calibrated as 30 gtts/ml.

$$\frac{X\,mL}{105\,gtt} = \frac{1\,mL}{30\,gtt} \qquad 30x = 105$$
$$x = 3.5\,mL/min$$

$$\frac{X\,min}{600\,mL} = \frac{1\,min}{3.5\,mL} \qquad 3.5x = 600$$
$$x = 171.43\,min$$

__171.43__ min

20. A 350 ml bag of D5W is running at 35 gtts/min using tubing calibrated to 10 gtts/ml. Calculate the total infusion time.

$$\frac{X\,mL}{35\,gtt} = \frac{1\,mL}{10\,gtt} \qquad 10x = 35$$
$$x = 3.5\,mL/min$$

$$\frac{X\,min}{350\,mL} = \frac{1\,min}{3.5\,mL} \qquad 3.5x = 350$$
$$x = 100\,min$$

__100__ min

Rx Success™ Complete Guide to Medical Math

In the following problems, solve for the amount of drug given per unit of time.

1. A 250 ml bag of NS contains 50 mg of drug. The IV is to be infused over two hours. How many mg/min of drug will the patient receive?

    $$\frac{X \text{ mg}}{1 \text{ min}} = \frac{50 \text{ mg}}{120 \text{ min}} \qquad 120x = 50 \qquad x = 0.42 \text{ mg/min}$$

    _____0.42_____ mg/min

2. A patient is to receive 40 mEq of potassium chloride in 250 ml of D5W over 4 hours. How many mEq of KCl will the patient receive every minute?

    $$\frac{X \text{ mEq}}{1 \text{ min}} = \frac{40 \text{ mEq}}{240 \text{ min}} \qquad 240x = 40 \qquad x = 0.17 \text{ mEq/min}$$

    _____0.17_____ mEq/min

3. A patient is to receive 1.5 g of drug in 250 mg of NS over 3 hours. How many mg of drug will the patient receive every minute?

    $$\frac{X \text{ mg}}{1 \text{ min}} = \frac{1500 \text{ mg}}{180 \text{ min}} \qquad 180x = 1500 \qquad x = 8.33 \text{ mg/min}$$

    _____8.33_____ mg/min

4. A 1200 ml bag of NS containing 75 U of regular insulin per liter, is to be infused over 6 hours. How many U of insulin will the patient receive per minute?

    $$\frac{X \text{ U}}{1 \text{ min}} = \frac{75 \text{ U}}{360 \text{ min}} \qquad 360x = 75 \qquad x = 0.21 \text{ U/min}$$

    _____0.21_____ U/min

5. A patient is to receive 2 grams of ampicillin in 500 ml of NS over 5 hours using 15 gtts/ml tubing. How many mg/min of ampicillin will the patient receive?

    $$\frac{X \text{ mg}}{1 \text{ min}} = \frac{2000 \text{ mg}}{300 \text{ min}} \qquad 300x = 2000 \qquad x = 6.67 \text{ mg/min}$$

    _____6.67_____ mg/min

Rx Success™ Complete Guide to Medical Math

6. A patient received an IV medication at a rate of 1.25 mg/min. After 112 minutes, how many mg of medication had the patient received?

$$\frac{X \text{ mg}}{112 \text{ min}} = \frac{1.25 \text{ mg}}{1 \text{ min}} \qquad X = 140 \text{ mg}$$

$$\frac{X \text{ mg}}{112 \text{ min}} = \frac{1.25 \text{ mg}}{1 \text{ min}}$$

$$X = 140 \text{ mg}$$

140 mg

7. A patient received an IV medication at a rate of 0.5 mg/min. How many mg will the patient receive after 3 hours?

$$\frac{X \text{ mg}}{180 \text{ min}} = \frac{0.5 \text{ mg}}{1 \text{ min}} \qquad X = 90 \text{ mg}$$

$$\frac{X \text{ mg}}{180 \text{ min}} = \frac{0.5 \text{ mg}}{1 \text{ min}}$$

$$X = 90 \text{ mg}$$

90 mg

8. A patient is to receive 500 ml of D5W containing 40,000 U of heparin to be infused at 2500 U/hr through microdrip tubing. How many ml of solution will the patient receive in 10 hours?

$$\frac{X \text{ mL}}{2500 \text{ U}} = \frac{500 \text{ mL}}{40000 \text{ U}} \qquad 40000X = 1250000$$

$$X = 31.25 \text{ mL/hr}$$

$$\frac{X \text{ mL}}{10 \text{ hr}} = \frac{31.25 \text{ mL}}{1 \text{ hr}} \qquad X = 312.50 \text{ mL}$$

312.5 ml

$$\frac{X \text{ mL}}{2500 \text{ U}} = \frac{500 \text{ mL}}{40000 \text{ U}}$$

$$40000X = 1250000$$

$$X = 31.25 \text{ mL/hr}$$

$$\times 10$$

$$312.5 \text{ mL}$$

Rx Success™ Complete Guide to Medical Math

Solve the following Advanced Drip Rate Calculations

1. A 450 ml bag of 5% Dextrose in Water contains 40 mEq of potassium chloride and is to run over six hours. Calculate how many mEq/min the patient is receiving.

    $$\frac{x\ mEq}{1\ min} = \frac{40\ mEq}{360\ min}$$
    $$360x = 40$$
    $$x = 0.11\ mEq/min$$

    $$\frac{x\ mEq}{1\ min} = \frac{40\ mEq}{360\ min}$$
    $$360x = 40$$
    $$x = 0.11\ mEq/min$$

    __0.11__ mEq/min

2. A 250 ml bag of fluid contains 500 mg of ciprofloxacin and is to be infused over two hours using microdrip tubing. Calculate how many mg/min of ciprofloxacin the patient is receiving.

    $$\frac{x\ mg}{1\ min} = \frac{500\ mg}{120\ min}$$
    $$120x = 500$$
    $$x = 4.17\ mg/min$$

    __4.17__ mg/min

3. A patient is to receive 800 mg of dopamine in 1000 ml of solution over six hours. How many mg of dopamine is the patient receiving every minute?

    $$\frac{x\ mg}{1\ min} = \frac{800\ mg}{360}$$
    $$360x = 800$$
    $$x = 2.22\ mg/min$$

    __2.22__ mg/min

4. A patient is to receive 0.2 mg/min of a drug using 15 gtts/ml tubing. The IV bag contains 250 ml of NS and 75 mg of drug. Calculate the flow rate in gtts/min.

    $$\frac{x\ mL}{0.2\ mg} = \frac{250\ mL}{75\ mg}$$
    $$75x = 50$$
    $$x = 0.67\ mL$$

    $$\frac{x\ gtt}{0.67\ mL} = \frac{15\ gtt}{1\ mL}$$
    $$x = 10.05\ gtts/min$$

    $$\frac{x\ mL}{0.2\ mg} = \frac{250\ mL}{75\ mg}$$
    $$75x = 50$$
    $$x = 0.67\ mL/min$$

    $$\frac{x\ gtt}{0.67\ mL} = \frac{15\ gtt}{1\ mL}$$
    $$x = 10\ gtt/min$$

    __10__ gtts/min

Rx Success™ Complete Guide to Medical Math

5. A 1000 ml bag of NS contains 25,000 units of heparin. The bag is running at 75 gtts/min using microdrip tubing. How many units of heparin is the patient receiving per minute? What is the total infusion time for the bag?

$$\frac{X\,mL}{75\,gtt} = \frac{1\,mL}{60\,gtt} \quad 60X = 75 \quad X = 1.25\,mL/min$$

$$\frac{X\,U}{1.25\,mL} = \frac{25000\,U}{1000\,mL} \quad 1000X = 31{,}250 \quad X = 31.25\,U/min$$

$$\frac{X\,min}{25000\,U} = \frac{1\,min}{31.25\,U} \quad 31.25X = 25000 \quad X = 800\,min$$

_____31.25_____ U/min

_____800_____ min

6. A 500 ml bag of 0.9% sodium chloride is running at 80 gtts/min through 12 gtts/ml tubing. The bag of fluid also contains 100 mEq of sodium bicarbonate. How many mEq of sodium bicarbonate is the patient receiving per minute?

$$\frac{X\,mL}{80\,gtt} = \frac{1\,mL}{12\,gtt} \quad 12X = 80 \quad X = 6.67\,mL/min$$

$$\frac{X\,mEq}{6.67\,mL} = \frac{100\,mEq}{500\,mL} \quad 500X = 667 \quad X = 1.33\,mEq/min$$

_____1.33_____ mEq/min

7. A 250 ml bag of D5W contains 1000 mg of drug to be infused over 90 minutes using 15 gtts/ml tubing. Calculate the flow rate in gtts/min. How many mg/min is the patient receiving?

$$\frac{X\,mL}{1\,min} = \frac{250\,mL}{90\,min} \quad 90X = 250 \quad X = 2.78\,mL/min$$

$$\frac{X\,gtt}{2.78\,mL} = \frac{15\,gtt}{1\,mL} \quad X = 41.7\,gtt/min$$

$$\frac{X\,mg}{2.78\,mL} = \frac{1000\,mg}{250\,mL} \quad 250X = 2780 \quad X = 11.12\,mg/min$$

_____42_____ gtts/min

_____11.11_____ mg/min

Rx Success™ Complete Guide to Medical Math

8. A patient is to receive 1.5 g of drug in 750 ml of Normal Saline. The IV is running at 95 gtts/min using 30 gtts/ml tubing. Calculate the total infusion time. How many mg/min of drug is the patient receiving?

$$\frac{x\ mL}{95\ gtt} = \frac{1\ mL}{30\ gtt} \qquad 30x = 95$$
$$x = 3.17\ mL/min$$

$$\frac{x\ min}{750\ mL} = \frac{1\ min}{3.17\ mL} \qquad 3.17x = 750$$
$$x = 236.59\ min$$

__236.59__ min

$$\frac{x\ mg}{3.17\ mL} = \frac{1500\ mg}{750\ mL} \qquad 750x = 4755$$
$$x = 6.34\ mg/min$$

__6.34__ mg/min

9. A patient is being administered 600 mg of clindamycin in 500 ml of D5W. The IV is currently running at 105 gtts/min. Calculate the total infusion time if the drop factor is 30 gtts/ml. How many mg of clindamycin is the patient receiving per minute?

$$\frac{x\ mL}{105\ gtt} = \frac{1\ mL}{30\ gtt} \qquad 30x = 105$$
$$x = 3.5\ mL/min$$

$$\frac{x\ min}{500\ mL} = \frac{1\ min}{3.5\ mL} \qquad 3.5x = 500$$
$$x = 142.86\ min$$

__142.86__ min

$$\frac{x\ mg}{3.5\ mL} = \frac{600\ mg}{500\ mL} \qquad 500x = 2100$$
$$x = 4.2\ mg/min$$

__4.2__ mg/min

10. A patient is to receive a 350 ml bag of D5W containing 75 mg of a drug. The IV is currently delivering 0.5 mg/min using tubing calibrated to 10 gtts/ml. Calculate the flow rate in gtts/min. Calculate the total infusion time.

$$\frac{x\ mL}{0.5\ mg} = \frac{350\ mL}{75\ mg} \qquad 75x = 175$$
$$x = 2.33\ mL/min$$

$$\frac{x\ gtt}{2.33\ mL} = \frac{10\ gtt}{1\ mL} \qquad x = 23.3\ gtts/min$$

__23__ gtts/min

$$\frac{x\ min}{350\ mL} = \frac{1\ min}{2.33\ mL} \qquad 2.33x = 350$$
$$x = 150.21\ min$$

__150.21__ min

Rx Success™ Complete Guide to Medical Math

11. A 1200 ml bag of NS containing 84 U of Regular insulin per liter, is to be infused over eight hours. The IV tubing is calibrated to deliver 20 gtts/ml. Calculate the flow rate in gtts/min. How many units of insulin will the patient receive every minute?

$$\frac{x\,mL}{1\,min} = \frac{1200\,mL}{480\,min} \quad 480x = 1200$$
$$x = 2.5\,mL/min$$

$$\frac{x\,gtt}{2.5\,mL} = \frac{20\,gtt}{1\,mL} \quad x = 50\,gtt/min$$

$$\frac{x\,U}{1200\,mL} = \frac{84\,U}{1000\,mL}$$
$$1000x = 100800$$
$$x = 100.8\,U$$

$$\frac{x\,U}{2.5\,mL} = \frac{100.8\,U}{1200\,mL} \quad 1200x = 252$$
$$x = 0.21\,U/min$$

__50__ gtts/min

__0.21__ U/min

12. A patient is to receive 800 ml of D5W containing 1200 mg of dopamine, through 15 gtts/ml tubing, to be infused over four hours. Calculate the flow rate in gtts/min. How many mg of dopamine will the patient receive every minute?

$$\frac{x\,mL}{1\,min} = \frac{800\,mL}{240\,min} \quad 240x = 800$$
$$x = 3.33\,mL/min$$

$$\frac{x\,gtt}{3.33\,mL} = \frac{15\,gtt}{1\,mL} \quad x = 49.95\,gtts/min$$

$$\frac{x\,mg}{3.33\,mL} = \frac{1200\,mg}{800\,mL} \quad 800x = 3996$$
$$x = 4.995\,mg/min$$

__50__ gtts/min

__5__ mg/min

13. A 500 ml bag containing 250 mg of vancomycin is running at 35 gtts/min through tubing calibrated to deliver 30 gtts/ml. How long will it take to infuse the entire bag? How many mg/min of vancomycin is the patient receiving?

$$\frac{x\,mL}{35\,gtt} = \frac{1\,mL}{30\,gtt} \quad 30x = 35$$
$$x = 1.17\,mL/min$$

$$\frac{x\,min}{500\,mL} = \frac{1\,min}{1.17\,mL} \quad 1.17x = 500$$
$$x = 427.35\,min$$

$$\frac{x\,mg}{1.17\,mL} = \frac{250\,mg}{500\,mL} \quad 500x = 292.50$$
$$x = 0.59\,mg/min$$

__427.35__ min

__0.59__ mg/min

14. An IV contains 0.4 mEq of KCl per ml of IV fluid. The patient is to receive 0.8 mEq of KCl per minute using microdrip tubing. Calculate the flow rate in gtts/min.

$$\frac{x\,mL}{0.8\,mEq} = \frac{1\,mL}{0.4\,mEq} \quad 0.4x = 0.8$$
$$x = 2\,mL/min$$

$$\frac{x\,gtt}{2\,mL} = \frac{60\,gtt}{1\,mL} \quad x = 120\,gtt/min$$

__120__ gtts/min

Rx Success™ Complete Guide to Medical Math

15. A 3.1 L bag of IV fluid contains 0.25 g of drug per liter. The IV is running at 45 gtts/min through tubing calibrated to deliver 10 gtts/ml. How many total mg are in the original IV bag? Calculate the total infusion time for the bag.

$$\frac{X\,g}{3.1\,L} = \frac{0.25\,g}{1\,L} \quad X = 0.775\,g \times 1000 = 775\,mg$$

$$\frac{X\,mL}{45\,gtt} = \frac{1\,mL}{10\,gtt} \quad 10X = 45 \quad X = 4.5\,mL/min$$

$$\frac{X\,min}{3100\,mL} = \frac{1\,min}{4.5\,mL} \quad 4.5X = 3100 \quad X = 688.89\,min$$

_____775_____ mg

_____688.89_____ min

16. A 250 ml bag of NS contains 1000 mg of dobutamine. The patient is to receive four mg of dopamine per minute using 15 gtts/ml tubing. Calculate the flow rate in gtts/min. Calculate the total infusion time for the IV.

$$\frac{X\,mL}{4\,mg} = \frac{250\,mL}{1000\,mg} \quad 1000X = 1000 \quad X = 1\,mL/min$$

$$\frac{X\,gtt}{1\,mL} = \frac{15\,gtt}{1\,mL} \quad X = 15\,gtts/min$$

$$\frac{X\,min}{250\,mL} = \frac{1\,min}{1\,mL} \quad X = 250\,min$$

_____15_____ gtts/min

_____250_____ min

17. A 2.4 L TPN contains 23 U of Regular insulin per liter of fluid. The TPN is running at 75 gtts/min using tubing calibrated at 20 gtts/ml. How many units of insulin is the patient receiving per min? How many total units of insulin were in the original TPN? Calculate the total infusion time for the IV.

2400 mL   1000 mL

$$\frac{X\,U}{2400\,mL} = \frac{23\,U}{1000\,mL} \quad 1000X = 55200 \quad X = 55.2\,U$$

$$\frac{X\,mL}{75\,gtt} = \frac{1\,mL}{20\,gtt} \quad 20X = 75 \quad X = 3.75\,mL/min$$

$$\frac{X\,U}{3.75\,mL} = \frac{55.2\,U}{2400\,mL} \quad 2400X = 207 \quad X = 0.09\,U/min$$

$$\frac{X\,min}{2400\,mL} = \frac{1\,min}{3.75\,mL} \quad 3.75X = 2400 \quad X = 640\,min$$

_____0.09_____ U/min

_____55.2_____ U

_____640_____ min

Rx Success™ Complete Guide to Medical Math

18. A patient is receiving 0.1 U of insulin per minute in a 500 ml IV containing a total of 65 units of regular insulin. The nurse is using IV tubing calibrated to deliver 12 gtts/ml. Calculate the total infusion time. Calculate the flow rate in gtts/min.

$$\frac{X\,mL}{0.1\,U} = \frac{500\,mL}{65\,U} \qquad \frac{X\,min}{65\,U} = \frac{1\,min}{0.1\,U} \qquad 0.1x = 65$$
$$x = 650\,min$$

$$65x = 50$$
$$x = 0.77\,mL/min \qquad \frac{X\,min}{500\,mL} = \frac{1\,min}{0.77\,mL} \qquad 0.77x = 500$$
$$x = 649.35\,min$$

$$\frac{X\,gtt}{0.77\,mL} = \frac{12\,gtt}{1\,mL} \qquad x = 9.24\,gtt/min$$

_____649_____ min

_____9_____ gtts/min

Chapter Thirteen

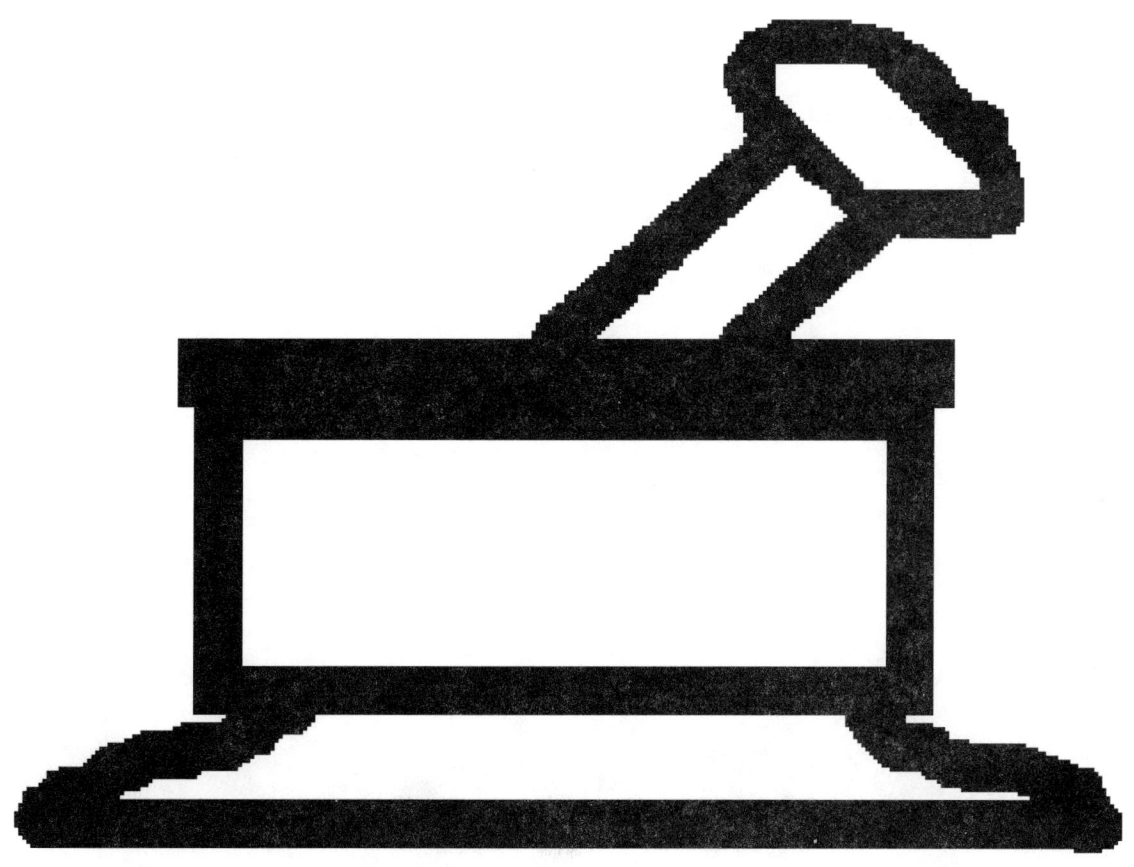

Alligations

Rx Success™ Complete Guide to Medical Math

Alligations

This particular skill is extremely valuable to health care providers. You will find it necessary to perform this calculation when a solution strength is ordered that is not commercially available or is not stocked by your facility. For instance, suppose a physician orders a 15% ascorbic acid solution. Upon checking the available stock, you discover that 10% and 25% solutions are available, but not a 15% solution. After completing this section, you should be able to combine proportional amounts of both 10% and 25% solutions to make the required volume of 15% solution.

Though these may seem like difficult calculations, alligations are no more difficult than making orange juice, or soup from a can! When making orange juice, for instance, you are instructed to add 3 cans of water for every one can of orange juice concentrate. This is a 3:1 ratio of water to concentrate. (3 parts water to 1 part orange juice concentrate).

Unlike canned orange juice and soup, pharmaceutical solutions do not provide a dilution ratio, so you must find your own. In the first Sample Problem we will take the ascorbic acid solution problem and find the ratio of 10% to 25% needed to formulate a 15% solution.

Read and study very carefully the Sample Problems that follow. When you feel comfortable with the technique used to perform alligations, move on to the Tutor Sheets™ and then the Homework at the end of the chapter.

Rx Success™ Complete Guide to Medical Math

Alligations – Sample Problems

1. **Calculate the ratio of solutions needed to make a 15% solution from 10% and 25% stock solutions.**

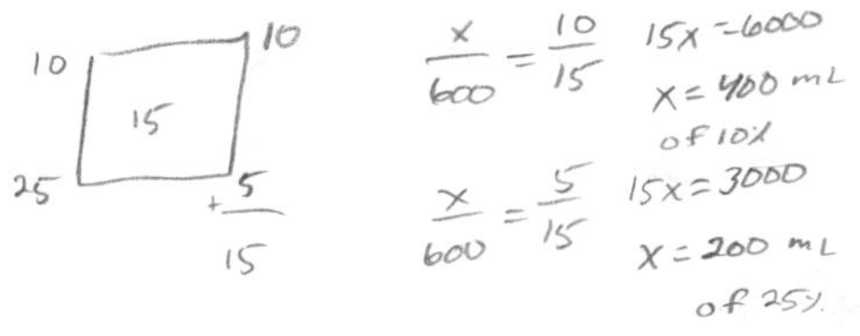

    First, identify the solution that has been ordered.

    Solution Ordered: 15%

    Now, identify the solutions that are available in stock.

    Solutions available in stock are 10% and 25%.

    The next step is to draw a checkerboard like the example provided below:

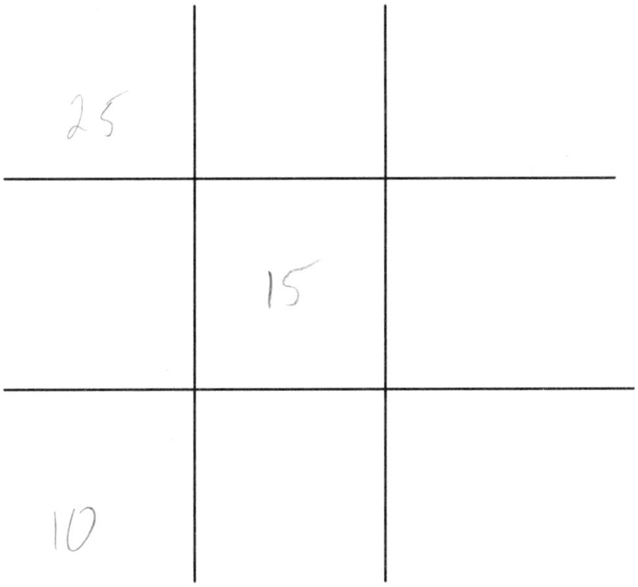

(handwritten work in margin:)
```
10        10
    15
25        5
    15
```
$$\frac{x}{600} = \frac{10}{15} \quad 15x = 6000 \quad x = 400 \text{ mL of 10%}$$
$$\frac{x}{600} = \frac{5}{15} \quad 15x = 3000 \quad x = 200 \text{ mL of 25%}$$

(checkerboard grid with:)
- 25 in top left
- 15 in center
- 10 in bottom left

To fill in the squares, follow these steps:

1. Write the percentage ordered in the middle square;

2. Write the highest percentage stock solution in the top left square;

3. Write the lowest percentage stock solution in the bottom left square.

Your checkerboard should now look like this:

25		
	15	
10		

4. Going down diagonally from the top left to the bottom right, subtract 15 from 25 and write your answer in the bottom right square.

5. Going up diagonally from the bottom left to the top right, subtract 10 from 15 and write your answer in the top right square.

Your checkerboard should now look like this:

25		5
	15	
10		10

6. Make a fraction out of your answers. Put the number in the top right square in the numerator (top) position. Now, put the number in the bottom right square in the denominator (bottom) position.

Rx Success™ Complete Guide to Medical Math

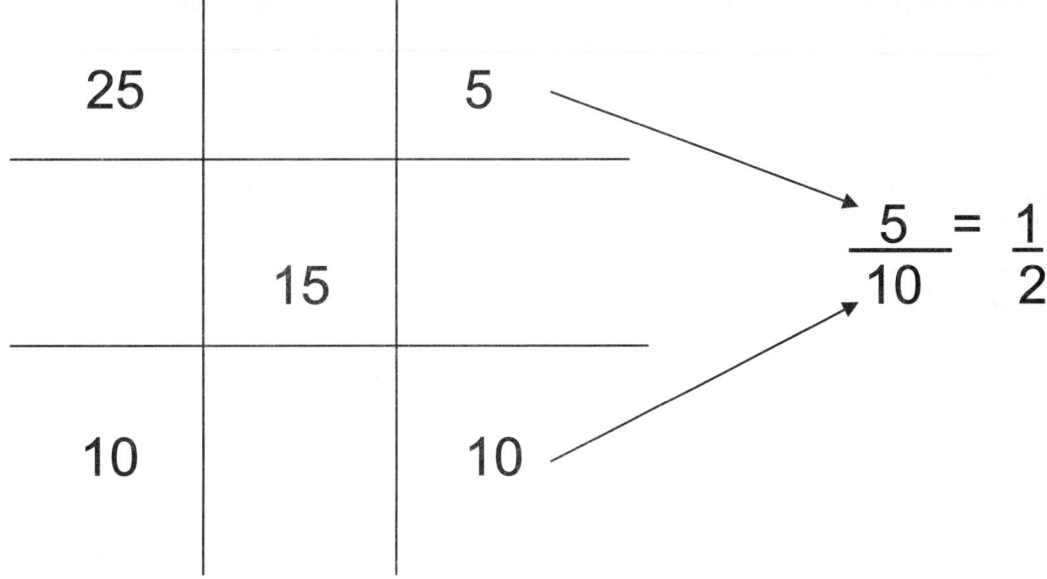

Reduce your faction to its lowest term.

    7. As you know, you can easily convert fractions to ratios by flipping the fraction on its side, one quarter turn counter clockwise.

       The fraction $\frac{1}{2}$ becomes the ratio 1:2

       The 1 (because it was the top number of the fraction) corresponds with the percent stock solution in the top left corner, and the 2 (because it was the bottom number of the fraction) corresponds with the percent stock solution in the bottom left corner.

       Our ratio now reads:

       1 part 25% solution to 2 parts 10% solution.

       If we were to make 3 cups of 15% ascorbic acid solution, we would combine one cup of 25% solution with 2 cups of 10% solution.

       Now that we have identified the proper ratio, we need to know how much of the solution to make. Let us suppose that the physician ordered 600 ml of the 15% solution. **How many ml of 25% and 10% solutions do we need to make 600 ml of a 15% solution?**

    8. Add the top and bottom numbers of your ratio (fraction) together.

       1 + 2 = 3

Rx Success™ Complete Guide to Medical Math

9. Take the answer you found in step 8 (which was 3 in this case) and divide it into the total number of ml needed (600 in this case).

   600 ÷ 3 = 200

10. Now, multiply the number you found in step nine by both the top and bottom numbers of the fraction found in step 6.

    In this case, it will look like this:

    $$\frac{1}{2} \times \frac{200}{200} = \frac{200}{400}$$

11. The top number of the fraction found in step 10 is the number of ml needed of the stock solution in the top left corner of your checkerboard (in this case, it is the 25% solution). The bottom number of the fraction denotes the number of ml needed of the stock solution in the bottom left corner of the checkerboard (in this case, it is the 10% solution).

    So, for our example, we find that we need:

    200 ml of the 25% ascorbic acid solution
    400 ml of the 10% ascorbic acid solution

    TO MAKE

    600 ml of a 15% ascorbic acid solution

    This may seem complex, but with some practice it will become an easy and helpful tool for you to use!

---

2. For this sample problem, the steps will not all be written out. If needed, refer to the previous problem.

   Order: 30% Solution. Need 250 ml.
   Stock: 15% Solution and 40% Solution

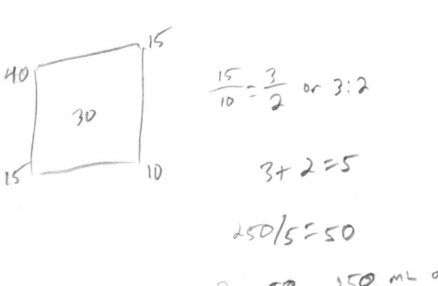

$\frac{x}{250} = \frac{15}{25}$ $25x = 3750$ $x = 150$ mL of 40%

$\frac{x}{250} = \frac{10}{25}$ $25x = 2500$ $x = 100$ mL of 15%

$\frac{15}{10} = \frac{3}{2}$ or 3:2

$3 + 2 = 5$

$250 / 5 = 50$

$\frac{3 \times 50}{2 \times 50} = \frac{150 \text{ mL of } 40\%}{100 \text{ mL of } 15\%}$

Rx Success™ Complete Guide to Medical Math

Set up the checkerboard, and find the fraction (ratio) needed for the problem.

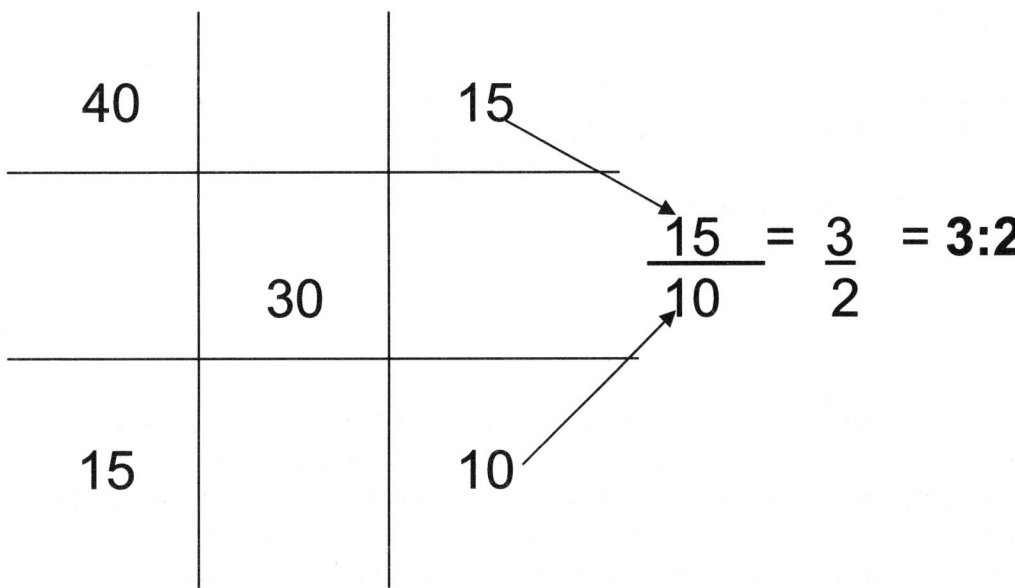

Add the two numbers of the ratio together and divide into the total number of mLs needed.

        a) 3 + 2 = 5
        b) 250 ÷ 5 = 50

Multiply 50 by both numbers of the fraction

$$\frac{3}{2} \times \begin{matrix} 50 \\ 50 \end{matrix} = \begin{matrix} 150 \\ 100 \end{matrix}$$

So, we need 150 ml of the 40% solution and 100 ml of the 15% solution to make 250 ml of a 30% solution.

**Note: When we speak of percent solutions, the percent number refers to the amount of drug in a solution; all else can be thought of as water. For instance, a 60% solution would be 60% drug and 40% water. So, water by itself is considered a 0% solution because it contains no drug.)

Rx Success™ Complete Guide to Medical Math

Alligations – Tutor Sheets™

USE THIS WORKSHEET AS A GUIDE TO HELP YOU SOLVE THE HOMEWORK PROBLEMS!

1. You receive an order to make 400 ml of a 7% solution from 5% and 10% stock solutions. How many ml of each stock solution do you need to compound this order?

   Handwritten work:
   $$\frac{X\,mL}{400\,mL} = \frac{2}{5} \quad 5x=800 \quad x=160\,mL\ of\ 10\%$$
   $$\frac{X\,mL}{400} = \frac{3}{5} \quad 5x=1200 \quad x=240\,mL\ of\ 5\%$$

   Step One – Identify the two stock solutions and write the percent strengths. Then, identify the percent strength and the amount (**in ml**) that you have been asked to make.

   Stock Soln #1 ___10___ %   Soln to be Made ___7___ %

   Stock Soln #2 ___5___ %   How many ml? ___400___ ml

   Step Two – Draw the alligation grid and correctly fill it in with the numbers you have identified from the problem.

   Grid (filled in):
   - Top left: 10
   - Top right: 2
   - Center: 7
   - Bottom left: 5
   - Bottom right: 3

   Handwritten work to right of grid:
   $$\frac{2}{3} = 2:3$$
   $$2+3=5 \quad 400/5 = 80$$
   $$2 \times 80 = 160\,mL\ of\ 10\%$$
   $$3 \times 80 = 240\,mL\ of\ 5\%$$

   Step Three – Find the ratio of stock solutions needed to compound the order. Continue working this problem to the right of the grid above.

   Step Four – Find the amounts of each stock solutions needed. Finish this problem to the right of the grid above.

Rx Success™ Complete Guide to Medical Math

2. Using a 50% amino acid solution and distilled water, you must make 1400 ml of a 37.5% amino acid solution. How many ml of each stock solution do you need to compound this order?

Step One – Identify the two stock solutions and write the percent strengths (be careful with the distilled water!). Then, identify the percent strength and the amount (**in ml**) that you have been asked to make.

Stock Soln #1 ___50___ %   Soln to be Made ___37.5___ %

Stock Soln #2 ___0___ %   How many ml? ___1400___ ml

Step Two – Draw the alligation grid and fill it in with the numbers you have identified from the problem.

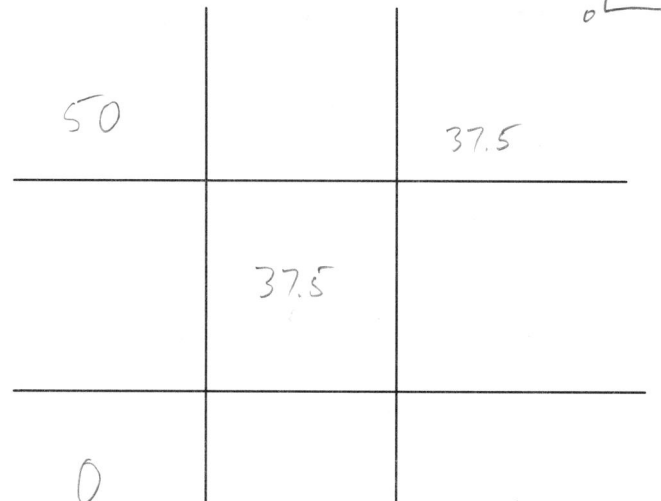

$\dfrac{x}{1400} = \dfrac{37.5}{50}$ $50x = 52500$ $x = 1050\,mL\text{ of }50\%$

$\dfrac{x}{1400} = \dfrac{12.5}{50}$ $50x = 17500$ $x = 350\,mL\text{ of distilled water}$

$\dfrac{37.5}{12.5} = \dfrac{3}{1} = 3:1$

$3 + 1 = 4$ $1400/4 = 350$

$3 \times 350 = 1050\,mL\text{ of }50\%$

$1 \times 350 = 350\,mL\text{ of water}$

50		37.5
	37.5	
0		12.5

Step Three – Find the ratio of stock solutions needed to compound the order. Continue working this problem to the right of the grid above.

Step Four – Find the amounts of each stock solutions needed. Finish this problem to the right of the grid above.

Rx Success™ Complete Guide to Medical Math

3. You receive an order to make 3.2 L of a 1.5% dextrose solution from 5% and 1% stock solutions. How many ml of each stock solution do you need to compound this order?

   Step One – Identify the two stock solutions and write the percent strengths. Then, identify the percent strength and the amount (**in ml**) that you have been asked to make.

   Stock Soln #1 ____5____ %   Soln to be Made ____1.5____ %

   Stock Soln #2 ____1____ %   How many ml? ____3200____ ml

   Step Two – Draw the alligation grid and fill it in with the numbers you have identified from the problem.

   ```
   5            0.5
       [1.5]
   1            3.5
   ```

   Grid (drawn):
   - Top-left: 5
   - Center: 1.5
   - Top-right: 0.5
   - Bottom-left: 1
   - Bottom-right: 3.5

   Work to the right of the grid:

   $5 \quad \boxed{} \quad 0.5$
   $\quad 1.5$
   $1 \quad \quad \underline{+3.5}$
   $\qquad\qquad 4.0$

   $\dfrac{x}{3200\,mL} = \dfrac{0.5}{4} \quad 4x = 1600 \quad x = 400\ mL\ of\ 5\%$

   $\dfrac{x}{3200\,mL} = \dfrac{3.5}{4} \quad 4x = 11200 \quad x = 2800\ mL\ of\ 1\%$

   $\dfrac{0.5}{3.5} = \dfrac{1}{7} = 1:7$

   $1 + 7 = 8 \qquad 3200/8 = 400$

   $1 \times 400 = 400\ mL\ of\ 5\%$
   $7 \times 400 = 2800\ mL\ of\ 1\%$

   Step Three – Find the ratio of stock solutions needed to compound the order. Continue working this problem to the right of the grid above.

   Step Four – Find the amounts of each stock solutions needed. Finish this problem to the right of the grid above.

Page - 239

Rx Success™ Complete Guide to Medical Math

4. You receive an order to make 280 ml of a 6% **amino acid** solution from a 10% **amino acid** solution and a 5% **Dextrose** solution. How many ml of each stock solution do you need to compound this order?

   Step One – Identify the two stock solutions and write the percent strengths. (**Hint: Think carefully about what number you should use for the 5% Dextrose solution. How much amino acid is in there?**) Then, identify the percent strength and the amount (**in ml**) that you have been asked to make.

   Stock Soln #1 __10__ %   Soln to be Made __6__ %

   Stock Soln #2 __0__ %   How many ml? __280__ ml

   Step Two – Draw the alligation grid and fill it in with the numbers you have identified from the problem.

10		6
	6	
0		4

   $\frac{6}{4} = \frac{3}{2} = 3:2$

   $3 + 2 = 5 \quad 280/5 = 56$

   $3 \times 56 = 168$ mL of 10%
   $2 \times 56 = 112$ mL of dextrose

   $\frac{X \text{ mL } 10\%}{280 \text{ mL total}} = \frac{6}{10}$ $10X = 1680$ $X = 168$ mL of 10%

   $\frac{X \text{ mL } 5\%}{280 \text{ mL total}} = \frac{4}{10}$ $10X = 1120$ $X = 112$ mL of Dextrose

   Step Three – Find the ratio of stock solutions needed to compound the order. Continue working this problem to the right of the grid above.

   Step Four – Find the amounts of each stock solutions needed. Finish this problem to the right of the grid above.

Answers to Tutor Sheets™ Calculations
1) 160 ml of 10%; 240 ml of 5%   2) 1050 ml of 50%; 350 ml of Distilled Water
3) 400 ml of 5%; 2800 ml of 1%   4) 168 ml of 10%; 112 ml of dextrose solution

Rx Success™ Complete Guide to Medical Math

Alligations - Homework

For the following problems, find:
a) the ratio needed (stronger solution listed first)
b) the amounts needed or each solution.

1. **Order:** 150 ml of 4% boric acid solution
   Stock: 2% and 10%

   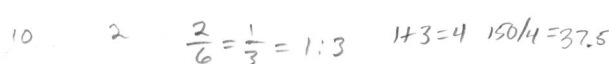

   Answers:
   a). Ratio Needed: ___1:3___.

   b). Amounts Needed: ___37.5 mL of 10%, 112.5 mL of 2%___.

2. **Order:** 700 ml of 40% dextrose solution
   Stock: 5% and 70%

   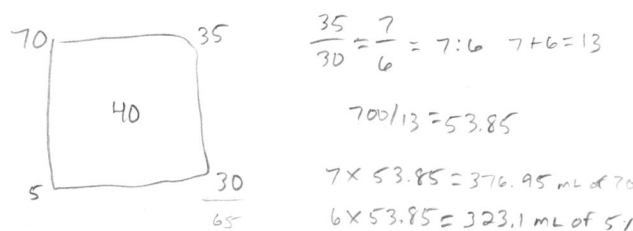

   Answers:
   a). Ratio Needed: ___7:6___.

   b). Amounts Needed: ___377 mL of 70% ; 323 mL of 5%___.

3. **Order:** 25 ml of 13% amino acid solution
   Stock: 11% and 15%

   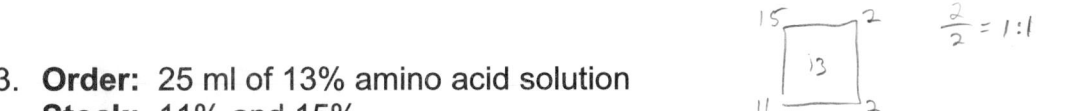

   Answers:
   a). Ratio Needed: ___1:1___.

   b). Amounts Needed: ___12.5 mL of 15% ; 12.5 mL of 11%___.

4. **Order:** 1500 ml of 4.5% boric acid solution
   Stock: 1.5% and 9%

   Answers:
   a). Ratio Needed: ___2:3___.

   b). Amounts Needed: ___600 mL of 9% , 900 mL of 1.5%___.

Rx Success™ Complete Guide to Medical Math

5. **Order:** 2800 ml of 5.5% ascorbic acid solution
   Stock: 2% and 10%

   Answers:
   a). Ratio Needed: __7:9__.

   b). Amounts Needed: __1225 mL of 10%, 1575 mL of 2%__.

6. **Order:** 1.3 L of 3% salt solution
   Stock: 5% and 2%

   Answers:
   a). Ratio Needed: __1:2__.

   b). Amounts Needed: __433 mL of 5%, 867 mL of 2%__.

7. **Order:** 0.75 L of 12.5% dextrose solution
   Stock: 70% and distilled water

   Answers:
   a). Ratio Needed: __5:23__.

   b). Amounts Needed: __134 mL of 70%, 616 mL of water__.

8. **Order:** 80 ml of 5% dextrose solution
   Stock: 70% and distilled water

   Answers:
   a). Ratio Needed: __1:13__.

   b). Amounts Needed: __6 mL of 70%, 74 mL of water__.

Rx Success™ Complete Guide to Medical Math

9. **Order:** 0.15 L of 1.2% ascorbic acid solution
   Stock: distilled water and 5%

   Answers:
   a). Ratio Needed: __6:19__.

   b). Amounts Needed: __36 mL of 5%, 114 mL of water__.

10. **Order:** 0.05 L of 0.5% salt solution
    Stock: 0.225% and 0.9%

    Answers:
    a). Ratio Needed: __11:16__.

    b). Amounts Needed: __20 mL of 0.9%, 30 mL of 0.225%__.

11. You are asked to make 630 ml of a 15% solution using 7% and 25% stock solutions. How many ml of each stock solution do you need? __280 mL of 25%, 350 mL of 7%__

12. You are asked to make 875 ml of a 4.5% stock solution. Your pharmacy stocks a 3% and an 8% solution. How many ml of 3% solution are needed? __612.5 mL of 3%__

13. The pharmacy stocks 150 ml bottles of a 35% amino acid solution, which is then diluted with distilled water. How many **bottles** are required to make 1400 ml of a 15% solution? __4 bottles__

$$\begin{array}{c} 35 \diagdown \diagup 15 \\ \boxed{15} \\ 0 \diagup \diagdown 20 \end{array}$$

$\dfrac{x}{1400} = \dfrac{15}{35}$ $35x = 21000$ $x = 600$ mL of 35%
$ \dfrac{600}{150} = 4$ bottles

$\dfrac{x}{1400} = \dfrac{20}{35}$ $35x = 28000$ $x = 800$ mL of water

Page - 243

Rx Success™ Complete Guide to Medical Math

14. You receive an order for 75 ml of a 1.5% solution. You need to use a 4% solution and distilled water to compound this order. How many ml of each will you need? *28 mL of 4%; 47 mL of water*

15. Using 70% and 5% stock solutions, you need to make 2500 ml of a 25% solution. How many ml of each stock solution are needed? *770 mL of 70%; 1730 mL of 5%*

16. A patient is to receive 750 ml of a 1.5% amino acid solution. The pharmacy stocks 15 ml ampules of an 80% amino acid solution, which you dilute with normal saline. How many ml of the 80% solution will you need? *14 mL of 80%*

17. Using 1000 ml stock bottles of a 15% dextrose solution and 250 ml stock bottles of a 70% dextrose solution, you are asked to make 4500 ml of a 25% dextrose solution. How many ml of each stock solution will you need? *819 mL of 70%; 3681 mL of 15%*

18. Using a 0.5% bacitracin irrigation solution and alcohol, how many ml of each are needed to compound 125 ml of a 0.05% bacitracin irrigation solution? *12.5 mL of 0.5%; 112.5 mL of alcohol*

Rx Success™ Complete Guide to Medical Math

19. Using a 70% dextrose solution and a 0.9% saline solution, you are asked to make 600 ml of a 50% dextrose solution. How many ml of each stock solution will you need to compound this order? 429 mL of 70% ; 171 mL of saline

20. You receive an order to make 80 ml of a 2.5% boric acid solution, using a 10% boric acid solution and 5% dextrose. How many ml of each solution will you need to compound this order? 20 mL of 10% ; 60 mL of dextrose

21. You are asked to make 360 g of a 0.05% hydrocortisone ointment using 5% hydrocortisone ointment and Aquaphor (as an ointment base). How many grams of each will you need to compound this order? 3.6 g of 5% ; 356.4 g of Aquaphor

$$\frac{x}{360} = \frac{0.05}{5} \quad 5x = 18 \quad x = 3.6 \text{ g of } 5\%$$

$$\frac{x}{360} = \frac{4.95}{5} \quad 5x = 1782 \quad x = 356.4 \text{ g of Aquaphor}$$

22. You receive an order for 1.5 lb of a 0.25% triamcinolone cream. You must make this compound using a 1% stock cream and Eucerin base, how many grams of each are needed? (1 lb = 454 g) 170 g of 1% ; 511 g of Eucerin

$$\frac{x \text{ g}}{1.5 \text{ lb}} = \frac{454 \text{ g}}{1 \text{ lb}} \quad x = 681 \text{ g}$$

$$\frac{x}{681} = \frac{0.25}{1} \quad x = 170.25 \text{ g of 1\% stock}$$

$$\frac{x}{681} = \frac{0.75}{1} \quad x = 510.75 \text{ g of Eucerin}$$

23. You receive an order for 3 L of a 5% bacitracin solution. To make this solution you will use a 6% bacitracin solution and sterile water. How many ml of sterile water do you need? 500 mL of water

Rx Success™ Complete Guide to Medical Math

24. How many ml of distilled water are needed to dilute a 2.5% saline solution down to 500 ml of normal saline? (hint: NS = 0.9%) 320 ml of water

25. How many ml of normal saline are needed to dilute a 70% dextrose solution down to 800 ml of a 5% dextrose solution? 743 ml of saline

Rx Success™ Complete Guide to Medical Math

Chapter Fourteen

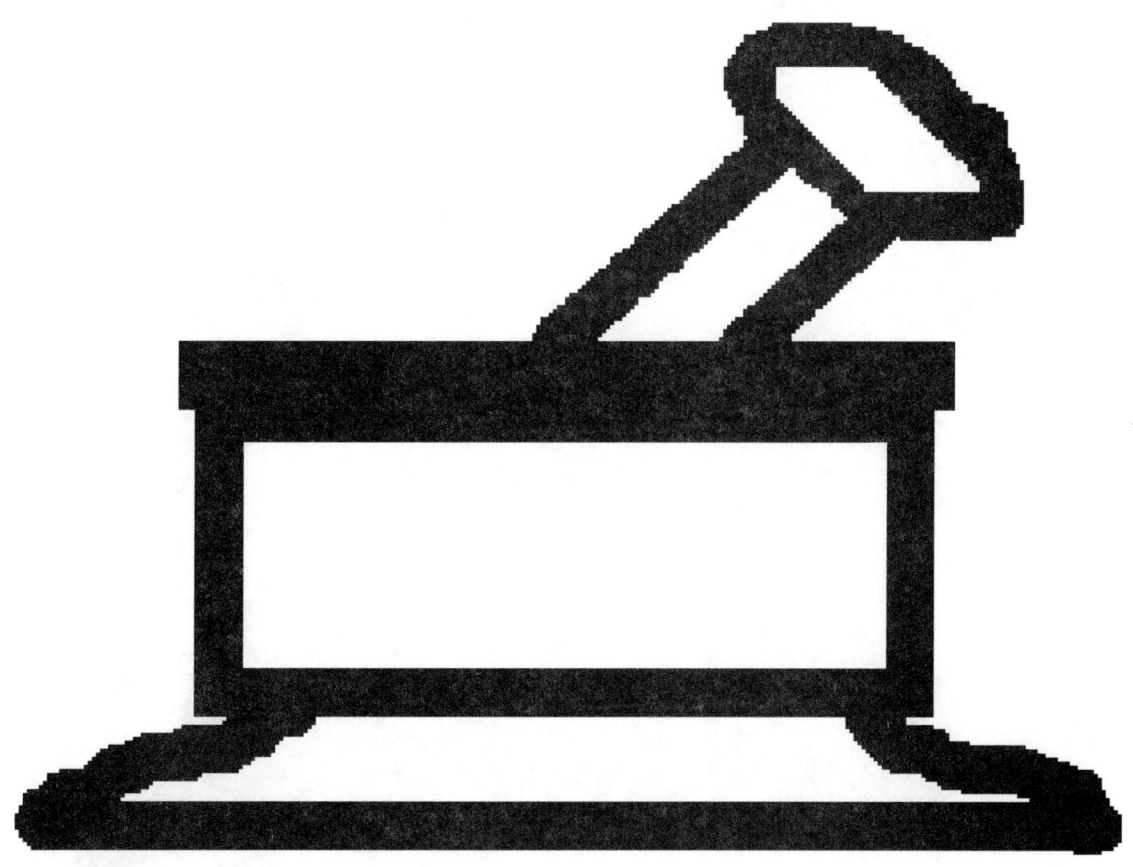

Pediatric Dosage Calculations

Rx Success™ Complete Guide to Medical Math

Pediatric Dosage Calculations

Many medications used for adults are also to treat infants and children. Although, the amounts of medication used in pediatric patients is certainly different than the amounts used for adults. Fortunately, there are several ways to determine the optimum doses for pediatric patients, based on individual information about each patient and sometimes usual adult dosage. This chapter will discuss several ways to determine a pediatric dose.

Clark's Rule

This formula is based on the child's weight in pounds. It takes into account the average weight for an adult, which is considered to be 150 lbs, and the average adult dose.

$$\frac{\text{child's weight (in lbs)}}{150 \text{ lb}} \times \text{adult dose} = \text{child's dose}$$

Cowling's Rule

This formula is based on the child's age in years and is not generally used. This formula is not an accurate way to calculate a patient's dose because there are so many other more important factors to take into consideration, than the patient's age.

$$\frac{\text{age at next birthday (in years)}}{24} \times \text{adult dose} = \text{child's dose}$$

Fried's Rule (children less than two years of age)

This formula is based on the child's age in months and is also rarely used. Fried's Rule should be limited to use on patients under two years old.

$$\frac{\text{child's age (in months)}}{150} \times \text{adult dose} = \text{child's dose}$$

Young's Rule (children two years or older)

This formula is also based on the child's age in years and is seen more frequently than Cowling's or Fried's formulas. Like Cowling's and Fried's Rule, this formula is not a very accurate way to calculate a patient's dose. However, you should be aware of this formula and know how to calculate doses based on Young's Rule.

Rx Success™ Complete Guide to Medical Math

$$\frac{\text{child's age (in years)}}{\text{child's age + 12 yrs}} \quad \text{X} \quad \text{adult dose} \quad = \quad \text{child's dose}$$

Using Body Surface Area

This is the most accurate way of determining pediatric dosages. The body surface area (BSA) of a patient takes into consideration both the height and weight of the patient. BSA may be calculated, however, most of the time a chart called a *nomogram* is used. A BSA is found on a nomogram by using a straight edge to draw a straight line between the patient's height measurement (in cm or in) and weight measurement (in lb or kg). The body surface area can be found where the line intersects the BSA column in the middle. Body surface area is measured in units of meters squared (m^2). Study the nomogram on the next page. The BSA has been determined for a child who is 24 inches tall and weighs 37 pounds. By positioning a ruler or straight edge at 24 inches on the left column and 37 pounds on the right column we are able to draw a straight line between the two points. The line we have drawn intersects the middle column at a BSA of 0.47 m^2. The formula for determining a pediatric dose based on BSA and the adult dose can be found below.

$$\frac{\text{child's BSA (in } m^2)}{1.73\ m^2} \quad \text{X} \quad \text{adult dose} \quad = \quad \text{child's dose}$$

Rx Success™ Complete Guide to Medical Math

Body Surface Area Nomogram

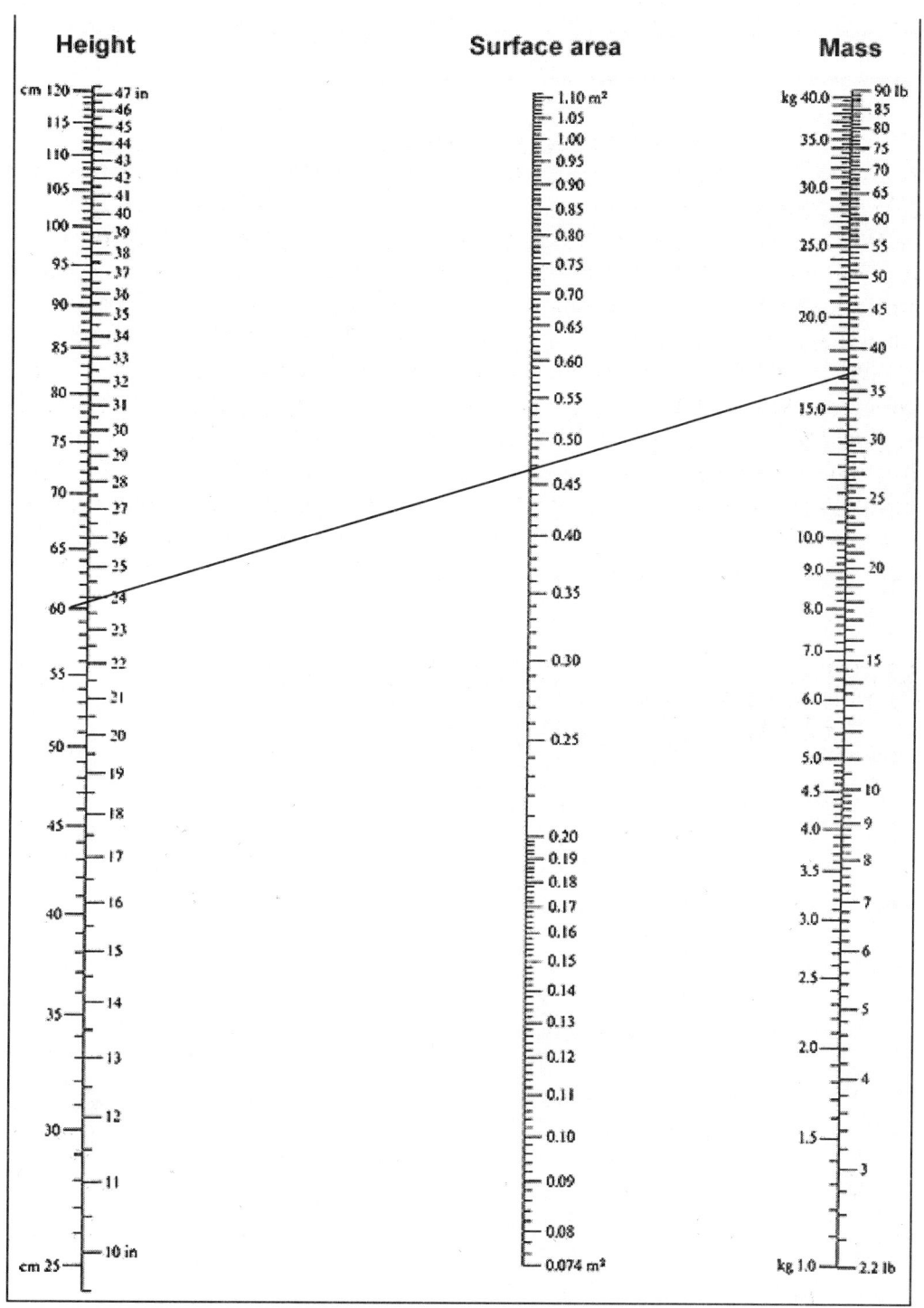

Rx Success™ Complete Guide to Medical Math

Pediatric Dosage Calculations - Sample Problems

Review the following sample problems and then move on to the Tutor Sheets™ and homework that follows.

1. A 10 year old, 68 lb child is to receive carbamazepine. The usual adult dose is 300 mg. Calculate the child's dose using Clark's Rule.

   $$\frac{\text{child's weight}}{\text{150 lb}} \times \text{adult dose} = \text{child's dose}$$

   Fill in the formula with the information from the problem. Then calculate the child's dose from the formula.

   $$\frac{\text{68 lb}}{\text{150 lb}} \times 300 \text{ mg} = \text{child's dose}$$

   First, divide 68 by 150 to get 0.45. Then multiply 0.45 by 300 to get a final answer of **135 mg**.

---

2. A 2 yr, 3 mos child who weighs 14 kg is to receive clarithromycin. The usual adult dosage is 500 mg. Calculate the child's dose using Fried's Rule.

   $$\frac{\text{child's age (in months)}}{150} \times \text{adult dose} = \text{child's dose}$$

   Find the patient's age in months (2 years = 24 mos + 3 mos = 27 mos). Fill in the formula with the information from the problem. Then calculate the child's dose from the formula.

   $$\frac{27 \text{ mo}}{150} \times 500 \text{ mg} = \text{child's dose}$$

   First, divide 27 by 150 to get 0.18. Then multiply 0.18 by 500 to get a final answer of **90 mg**.

---

3. The usual adult dosage for IV famotidine is 20 mg every 12 hours. Calculate a pediatric dose for a 23 kg, 3 year old child using Young's Rule.

   $$\frac{\text{child's age (in years)}}{\text{child's age + 12 yrs}} \times \text{adult dose} = \text{child's dose}$$

   Fill in the formula with the information from the problem. Then calculate the child's dose from the formula.

$$\frac{3 \text{ yr}}{15 \text{ yr}} \quad X \quad 20 \text{ mg} \quad = \quad \text{child's dose}$$

First, divide 3 by 15 to get 0.2. Then multiply 0.2 by 20 to get a final answer of **4 mg**.

---

4. A 16 month old infant is 27 inches in length and weighs 10 kg. Calculate the dose of a medication where the adult dose is 750 mg. Use the nomogram and the child's BSA to determine the child's correct dose.

$$\frac{\text{child's BSA (in m}^2\text{)}}{1.73 \text{ m}^2} \quad X \quad \text{adult dose} \quad = \quad \text{child's dose}$$

Find the patient's BSA by using the nomogram on page 251 by drawing a line between the patient's height and weight. The patient's BSA can be found in the middle column at the intersection of the line. Fill in the formula with the patient's BSA. Then calculate the child's dose from the formula.

$$\frac{0.41 \text{ m}^2}{1.73 \text{ m}^2} \quad X \quad 750 \text{ mg} \quad = \quad \text{child's dose}$$

First, divide 0.41 by 1.73 to get 0.24. Then multiply 0.24 by 750 to get a final answer of **180 mg**.

Rx Success™ Complete Guide to Medical Math

Pediatric Dosage Calculations – Tutor Sheets™

USE THIS WORKSHEET AS A GUIDE TO HELP YOU SOLVE THE HOMEWORK PROBLEMS!

1. Using Young's Rule, calculate the dosage of a medication for a 4 year old child who weighs 37 pounds. The normal adult dose of this drug is 175 mg.

   Step One: Write out the formula that you need to solve the problem.

   $$\frac{\text{child's age (in years)}}{\text{child's age + 12 yrs}} \times \text{adult dose} = \text{child's dose}$$

   Step Two: Fill in the formula with the information from the problem.

   _____ X _____ = _____ mg

   Final Answer: ___43.75___ mg

---

2. Using Clark's Rule, calculate the amount of drug needed for one dose for an 18 month old child who weighs 26 pounds. The usual adult dose is 700 mg per day in four equally divided doses.

   Step One: Write out the formula that you need to solve the problem.

   $$\frac{\text{child's weight}}{150 \text{ lb}} \times \text{adult dose} = \text{child's dose}$$

   Step Two: Fill in the formula with the information from the problem.

   _____ X _____ = _____ mg

   Step Three: The problem said the adult dose is **per day** in four equally divided doses. This means that the answer to step 2 must be divided by four to get the amount of drug needed for one dose.

   _____ divided by 4 = _____ mg

   Final Answer: ___30.33___ mg

Rx Success™ Complete Guide to Medical Math

3. A 10 year old child weighs 75 lb and is 46 in tall. Using the body surface area calculation, calculate a dose for this patient if the usual adult dose is 215 mg.

   Step One: Write out the formula that you need to solve the problem.

   $$\frac{\text{child's BSA (in m}^2)}{1.73 \text{ m}^2} \times \text{adult dose} = \text{child's dose}$$

   Step Two: Use the BSA Nomogram and the child's height and weight to determine the child's BSA.

   Child's BSA = _____ m²

   Step Three: Fill in the formula with the information from the problem.

   _____ X _____ = _____mg

---

4. A 45 lb child who is 2 ft 5 in tall is ordered to receive 25 mg q8h of a drug. The normal adult dose must not exceed 150 mg per day. Using the BSA calculation, determine if the pediatric dose is safe.

   Step One: Write out the formula that you need to solve the problem.

   $$\frac{\text{child's BSA (in m}^2)}{1.73 \text{ m}^2} \times \text{adult dose} = \text{child's dose}$$

   Step Two: Use the BSA Nomogram to determine the child's BSA.

   Child's BSA = _____ m²

   Step Three: Fill in the formula with the information from the problem.

   _____ X _____ = _____mg
   max dose per day

   Step Four: The pediatric dose calculated in step three is the max dose that the child can receive per day. Since the ordered dose requires the child to receive 25 mg every 8 hours they will receive a total of *three doses* in one day. Therefore to determine the safety of the child's dose we must multiply 25 mg by three. Then compare this amount of drug to the answer in step three.

   _____ X _____ = _____mg
   ordered dose per day

   Final Answer (circle one): Is the dose safe?   Yes   No

Answers to Tutor Sheets™ Calculations
1) 43.75 mg   2) 30.33 mg   3) 123.03 mg   4) No

Rx Success™ Complete Guide to Medical Math

Pediatric Dosage Calculations - Homework

Follow the instructions to calculate the following pediatric dosages using the formulas from the previous section.

1. The adult dose of a drug is 1250 mg every 12 hours. Calculate a pediatric dose for a 6 year old child who weighs 47 pounds using Clark's Rule.

$$\frac{47}{150} \times 1250 = 392 \text{ mg}$$

2. Using Fried's Rule, calculate the pediatric dosage for a 2 year old patient who weighs 24 pounds. The average adult dose of the ordered medication is 300 mg.

$$\frac{24}{150} \times 300 = 48 \text{ mg}$$

3. Calculate the pediatric dose for a child who weighs 36 lbs. The average adult dose is 175 mg. Use Clark's Rule to determine the pediatric dose.

$$\frac{36}{150} \times 175 = 42 \text{ mg}$$

4. Using Young's Rule, calculate a dose for a 6 yr old child who weighs 43 lbs. The average adult dose is 75 mg.

$$\frac{6}{18} \times 75 = 25 \text{ mg}$$

5. If the usual adult dosage for an injectable drug is 375 mg, calculate a pediatric dose for a 13 kg, 3 year old child using Young's Rule.

$$\frac{3}{15} \times 375 = 75 \text{ mg}$$

Rx Success™ Complete Guide to Medical Math

6. The usual adult dosage for IV furosemide is 80 mg. Calculate a pediatric dose for an 11 yr old child who weighs 82 lb using Cowling's Rule.

$$\frac{12}{24} \times 80 = 40 \text{ mg}$$

7. Using Fried's Rule, calculate a pediatric dose for a 14 month old child. The average adult dose is 50 mg.

$$\frac{14}{150} \times 50 = 4.67 \text{ mg}$$

8. The usual adult dosage of a drug is 400 mg. Calculate a pediatric dose for a 4 ½ yr old child who weighs 17 kg using Cowling's Rule.

$$\frac{5}{24} \times 400 = 83 \text{ mg}$$

9. Calculate a pediatric dose for a 10 yr old child who weighs 35 kg using Young's Rule. The usual adult dosage is 225 mg.

$$\frac{10}{22} \times 225 = 102.27 \text{ mg}$$

10. If the normal adult dose of a drug is 750 mg, calculate a pediatric dose for an 8 yr old child who weighs 29 kg, using Clark's Rule.

$$\frac{x \text{ lb}}{29 \text{ kg}} = \frac{2.2 \text{ lb}}{1 \text{ kg}}$$

$$x = 63.8 \text{ lbs}$$

$$\frac{63.8}{150} \times 750 = 319 \text{ mg}$$

11. Using Fried's Rule, calculate the dosage of penicillin when the adult dosage is 50,000 U. The patient is 18 months old and weighs 29 lbs.

$$\frac{18}{150} \times 50000 = 6000 \text{ U}$$

12. If the usual adult dose of tetracycline is 250 mg, calculate a pediatric dose for an 8 month old child who weighs 10 kg. Use Clark's Rule to determine the correct dose.

$$\frac{x \text{ lb}}{10 \text{ kg}} = \frac{2.2 \text{ lb}}{1 \text{ kg}}$$

$$x = 22 \text{ lb}$$

$$\frac{22}{150} \times 250 = 36.67 \text{ mg}$$

13. The usual adult dose of ASA is 10 grains. Using Clark's Rule, calculate how many grains you would administer to a 28 month old child who weighs 13.8 kg.

$$\frac{x \text{ lb}}{13.8 \text{ kg}} = \frac{2.2 \text{ lb}}{1 \text{ kg}}$$

$$x = 30.36 \text{ lb}$$

$$\frac{30.36}{150} \times 10 = 2 \text{ gr}$$

14. If the normal adult dose of a drug is 750 mg, calculate a pediatric dose for a 4 yr old child who weighs 21 kg and is 40 inches tall, using Cowling's Rule.

$$\frac{5}{24} \times 750 = 156.25 \text{ mg}$$

15. If the normal adult dose of a drug is 1500 mg, calculate a pediatric dose for an 18 month old child who weighs 15 kg, using Clark's Rule.

$$\frac{x \text{ lb}}{15 \text{ kg}} = \frac{2.2 \text{ lb}}{1 \text{ kg}}$$

$$x = 33 \text{ lb}$$

$$\frac{33}{150} \times 1500 = 330 \text{ mg}$$

16. Calculate a safe oral dosage of digoxin for a 45 lb, 5 year old child, using Young's Rule. The normal adult, oral dose is 0.25 mg.

$$\frac{5}{17} \times 0.25 \text{ mg} = 0.07 \text{ mg}$$

17. How many mg of atropine should be given to a 3 month old infant if the usual adult dosage is 0.4 mg. Use Fried's rule to calculate this dose.

$$\frac{3}{150} \times 0.4 = 0.008 \text{ mg}$$

Rx Success™ Complete Guide to Medical Math

Use the nomogram that follows, or the body surface areas given in the problems, to calculate the correct pediatric dosages.

Height	Surface area	Mass
cm 25 – 120 cm (10 in – 47 in)	0.074 m² – 1.10 m²	kg 1.0 – 40.0 kg (2.2 lb – 90 lb)

Rx Success™ Complete Guide to Medical Math

18. A child's body surface area is 0.42 m². Calculate a dose for this child if the normal adult dose is 80 mg.

$$\frac{0.42}{1.73} \times 80 = 19.42 \text{ mg}$$

19. A child's BSA is 0.51 m². Calculate a normal dose for this child if the normal adult dose is 1200 mg.

$$\frac{0.51}{1.73} \times 1200 = 353.76 \text{ mg}$$

20. Calculate the pediatric dose of cephalexin for a child whose BSA is 0.6 m². The usual adult dose is 500 mg.

$$\frac{0.6}{1.73} \times 500 = 173.41 \text{ mg}$$

21. The patient is a child who is 3 ft, 4 in tall. The child weighs 37 lbs. Calculate the correct dose for this patient, using the body surface area calculation. The normal adult dose for the drug is 150 mg.

$$\frac{0.68}{1.73} \times 150 = 58.96 \text{ mg}$$

22. A 9 year old child who weighs 68 lb is 4 ft tall. Using the body surface area calculation, calculate a dose for this patient if the usual adult dose is 215 mg.

$$\frac{1.02}{1.73} \times 215 = 126.76 \text{ mg}$$

23. Calculate a pediatric dose if the adult dose is 500 mg. The patient is a 4 year old child who weighs 20 kg and is two feet tall.

$$\frac{x \text{ lb}}{20 \text{ kg}} = \frac{2.2 \text{ lb}}{1 \text{ kg}}$$
$$x = 44 \text{ lb}$$

$$\frac{0.50}{1.73} \times 500 = 144.51 \text{ mg}$$

Rx Success™ Complete Guide to Medical Math

24. Calculate a dose for a 6 year old child. The patient weighs 22 kg and is 114 cm tall. The normal adult dose is 1500 mg.

25. Calculate the dosage of a drug for a 23 lb child who is 20 months old and 32 inches long. The normal adult dosage for this drug is 300 mg.

26. A 13 year old adolescent stands 5 ft 2 in tall with a BSA of 1.15 m². Calculate a dose for this patient if the normal adult dose is 50 mg every 6 hours.

$$\frac{1.15}{1.73} \times 50 = 33.24 \text{ mg}$$

27. A 9 year old child who is 4 ft tall and weighs 68 lbs is ordered to receive 520 mg of a drug. Is this the correct dose if the normal adult dose is 900 mg?

28. An 8 month old child is ordered to receive 15 mg of a drug every 6 hours. The child weighs 11 lb and is 19 inches long. If the normal adult dose is 450 mg per day, does the child's ordered dose exceed the daily limit, based on the body surface area?

Rx Success™ Complete Guide to Medical Math

29. A 28 month old child is ordered to receive 500 mg of a drug every day. The child weighs 25 kg and is 90 cm long. If the normal adult dose is 800 mg per day, does the child's ordered dose exceed the daily limit, based on the body surface area?

30. A 12 year old child is ordered to receive 400 mg of carbenacillin IM. The child weighs 90 lb and is 46.5 in tall. If the normal adult dose is 500 mg IM, determine if the ordered dose for the child is safe.

Advanced Pediatric Dosage Calculations (please refer back to the nomogram on page 260 if necessary).

31. A 5 year old child is ordered to receive 100 mg of a drug every 12 hours. The usual adult dosage is between 500 mg and 750 mg per day. Using Young's Rule, determine if the ordered dose for this child is appropriate.

$$\frac{5}{17} \times 500 = 147.06 \text{ mg}$$

$$\frac{5}{17} \times 750 = 220.59 \text{ mg}$$

$100 \times 2 = 200/\text{day}$

So Yes

32. A 19 lb child is ordered to receive 250 mg q6h of a drug. The normal adult dose for this drug is between 800 mg and 1200 mg per day in four equally divided doses. Using Clark's Rule, determine if the order is correct.

$$\frac{19}{150} \times 800 = 101.33 \text{ mg}$$

$$\frac{19}{150} \times 1200 = 152 \text{ mg}$$

$250 \times 4 = 1000 \text{ mg/day}$

So No

33. A 34.1 kg child has been ordered to receive 25 mg of cefuroxime three times daily. The package insert gives the following dosing parameters for adults: Administer between 100 and 150 mg/kg/day in equally divided doses every 8 hours. Using Clark's Rule, determine if the pediatric dose amount is correct.

$$\frac{x \text{ mg}}{34.1 \text{ kg}} = \frac{100 \text{ mg}}{1 \text{ kg}} \quad x = 3410 \text{ mg/day}$$

$$\frac{x \text{ mg}}{34.1 \text{ kg}} = \frac{150 \text{ mg}}{1 \text{ kg}} \quad x = 5115 \text{ mg/day}$$

$$\frac{x \text{ lb}}{34.1 \text{ kg}} = \frac{2.2 \text{ lb}}{1 \text{ kg}}$$

$x = 75.02 \text{ lb}$

$$\frac{75.02}{150} \times 100 = 50.01 \text{ mg}$$

$$\frac{75.02}{150} \times 150 = 75.02 \text{ mg}$$

$25 \times 3 = 75$

So Yes

34. A 12 kg child has been ordered to receive 150 mg of a drug every four hours. The usual adult dosage must not exceed 2.5 g per day. Using Clark's Rule, determine whether or not the child's dose exceeds the maximum limit.

$$\frac{x \text{ lb}}{12 \text{ kg}} = \frac{2.2 \text{ lb}}{1 \text{ kg}}$$

$$x = 26.4 \text{ lb}$$

$$\frac{26.4}{150} \times 2500 = 440 \text{ mg}$$

$150 \times 6 = 900$ mg

so

Exceeds Max

35. A 12 kg child has been ordered to receive 0.05 g of a drug every six hours. The usual adult dosage must not exceed 750 mg every 12 hours. Using Clark's Rule, determine whether or not the child's dose exceeds the maximum limit.

132 mg

36. A 6 year old child who weighs 50 lbs and is 3 feet 11 inches tall is to receive 100 mg of a drug every 12 hours. The recommended adult dose is 500 mg per day in two, equally divided doses. Using the body surface area calculation, determine whether or not the child's dose exceeds the recommendations.

37. A 16 month old child who weighs 10 kg is 28 inches long is to receive 0.75 mg of a drug every 2 hours. The adult dose may not exceed 50 mg per day. Using the body surface area calculation, determine whether or not the child's dose exceeds the recommendations.

38. Calculate the correct daily dosage range for a 28 month old child who weighs 26 lb and is 35 inches in length. The adult dosage range is 500 mg to 750 mg per day in equally divided doses given every 8 hours.

Rx Success™ Complete Guide to Medical Math

Chapter Fifteen

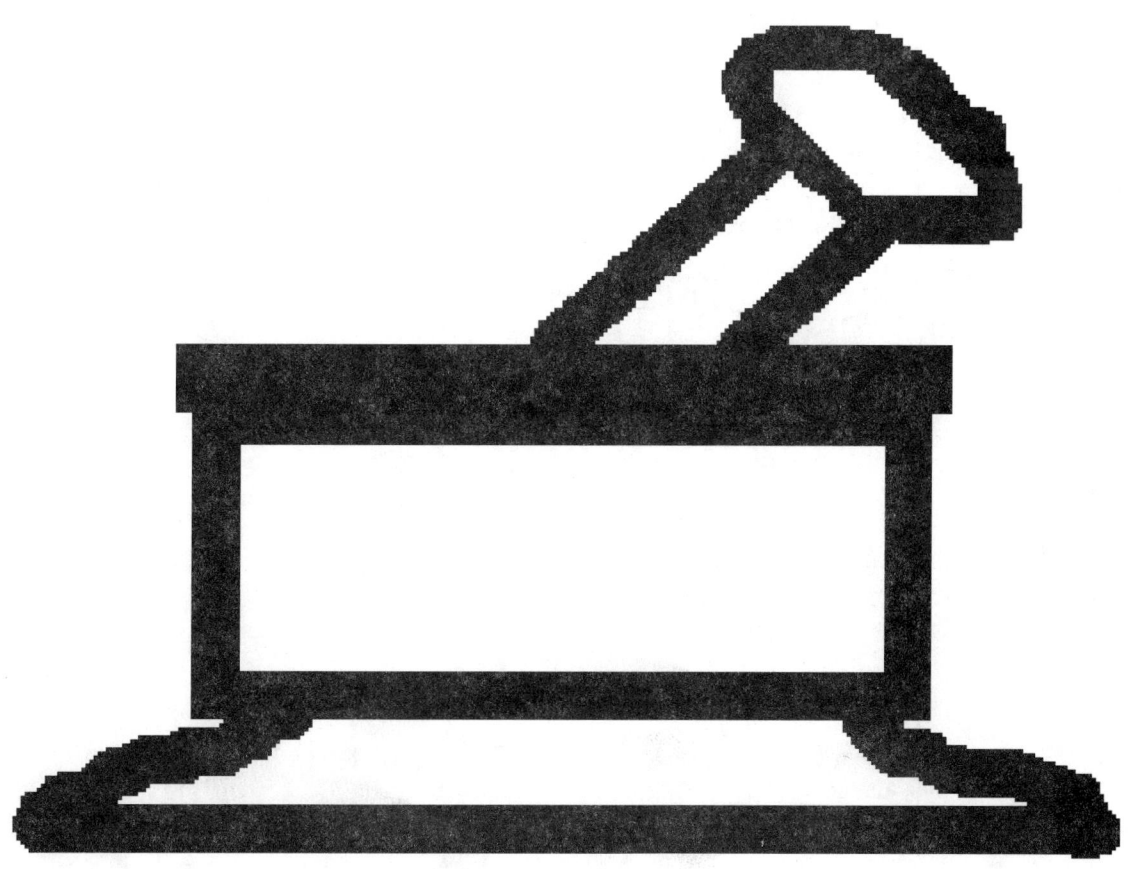

Pharmaco-Economic Calculations

Rx Success™ Complete Guide to Medical Math

Pharmaco-Economics

Before getting started on this section, familiarize yourself with the following terms and formulas. Refer back to these economic definitions and formulas to complete the sample problems and homework that follows.

TERMS:

1. **AWP** – An acronym that stands for "average wholesale price".

2. **Markup** (also called "**Gross Profit**") – This is the difference between the retail selling price and the wholesale cost. This value is an actual dollar amount.

3. **Markup Percentage** (or **Percent Markup**) – This is the percentage that a pharmacy uses to determine the markup amount.

4. **Overhead** – This is the amount of all of the costs incurred in operating the pharmacy (see page 245 for a sample list of overhead expenses). A portion of the markup for each drug is used to pay for overhead expenses.

5. **Professional Fee** – This is a flat fee that a pharmacy will usually add to the retail price of every prescription. Most pharmacies will also use this amount as the minimum prescription charge. The professional fee must be added **after** the markup.

6. **Profit** (also called "**Net Profit**") – This is the portion of the markup amount that is left after the overhead has been subtracted. Simply put, it is profit *after* expenses.

7. **Retail** (also called "**Selling Price**") – This is the price the consumer pays for a product. A pharmacy will add a markup amount to the wholesale price to calculate the retail price.

8. **Wholesale** (also called "**Acquisition Cost**" or simply "**Cost**") – This is the price that a wholesaler charges a retailer. The pharmacy pays wholesale prices for its products.

Rx Success™ Complete Guide to Medical Math

Pharmaco-Economics Formulas

All of the following formulas include algebraic variations. Use this page to pick the correct formula or formula variation, based on the information given in your problem.

1. **Retail (Selling Price) = Wholesale + Markup**

    ➤ **Wholesale = Retail – Markup**

    ➤ **Markup = Retail – Wholesale**

2. **Markup = Overhead + Profit**

    ➤ **Overhead = Markup – Profit**

    ➤ **Profit = Markup – Overhead**

3. **Markup Percentage = $\dfrac{\text{Markup}}{\text{Wholesale}} \times 100$**

    or, Markup ÷ Wholesale × 100

    ➤ **Markup = $\dfrac{\text{Markup Percentage} \times \text{Wholesale}}{100}$**

    ➤ **Wholesale = $\dfrac{\text{Markup}}{\text{Markup Percentage}} \times 100$**

**NOTE: The completion of some problems require several formulas, used in succession. For instance, you may have to calculate the markup separately before adding it to the wholesale price to obtain the retail price.

Rx Success™ Complete Guide to Medical Math

Pharmacoeconomics is an area of medical math that is extremely important to Pharmacy Technicians and their employers. A pharmacy must make money in order to retain employees. If a pharmacy were to sell products to consumers without first marking it up, they could no longer afford to pay employee salaries. Besides the cost of employees, there are numerous other expenses that must be paid. Here are a few

a) Electricity
b) Water
c) Housekeeping
d) Rent
e) Liability Insurance
f) Computer Maintenance and Software Updates
g) Reference Books
h) Drug Inventory
i) Office Supplies (pens, paper clips, bags, vials, etc.)
j) Telephone

All of these expenses incurred by a pharmacy, including pharmacist and technician salaries, are called **overhead**. Every item sold by a pharmacy must share the burden of overhead.

If a pharmacy were to determine the **retail** price by adding **overhead** to the **wholesale** price, there would be no **profit**. As you know, a business must be profitable to survive. Therefore, in addition to **wholesale** price and **overhead**, a pharmacy must determine how much **profit** they wish to make. **Profit** and **overhead** added together is called **markup**.

Overhead + Profit = Markup

Once you have calculated the **markup**, add it to the **wholesale** price to get the **retail** price.

Markup + Wholesale = Retail

You may also combine both formulas to get:

Overhead + Profit + Wholesale = Retail

Look at the following sample problems and then do the homework problems at the end of this section.

Rx Success™ Complete Guide to Medical Math

Pharmaco-Economics - Sample Problems

1. XYZ Wholesaler sells aspirin to ABC Pharmacy for the wholesale price of $0.38 per bottle. ABC Pharmacy must charge $0.15 for overhead and would like to make a profit of $0.10 on each bottle of aspirin. **Calculate the total markup and the retail price for the aspirin.**

   Known Values

   Wholesale = $0.38
   Overhead = $0.15
   Profit = $0.10

   a) Calculate the markup using the following formula.

   Markup = Overhead + Profit

   Markup = $0.15 + $0.10

   Markup = $0.25

   b) Calculate the retail price using the following formula.

   Retail = Wholesale + Markup

   Retail = $0.38 + $0.25

   Retail = $0.63

---

2. ABC Pharmacy pays $327.63 per case for a new biotech drug. The overhead assigned to this drug is $52.97 per case. The pharmacy would like to make $37.29 profit per case. **Calculate the total markup and the retail price (per case).**

   Known Values

   Wholesale = $327.63
   Overhead = $52.97
   Profit = $37.29

Rx Success™ Complete Guide to Medical Math

    a) Calculate the markup using the following formula.

        Markup = Overhead + Profit

        Markup = $52.97 + $37.29

        Markup = $90.26

    b) Calculate the retail price using the following formula.

        Retail = Wholesale + Markup

        Retail = $327.63 + $90.26

        Retail = $417.89

---

3. The markup on pantyhose at ABC Pharmacy is $1.37. The overhead is $0.75. The pharmacy pays XYZ Wholesaler $0.97 for each pair. **Calculate the pharmacy's profit and the retail selling price on each pair.**

<u>Known Values</u>

Markup = $1.37
Overhead = $0.75
Wholesale = $0.97

    a) Calculate the profit using the following formula.

        Profit = Markup - Overhead

        Profit = $1.37 - $0.75

        Profit = $0.62

    b) Calculate the retail price using the following formula.

        Retail = Wholesale + Markup

        Retail = $0.97 + $1.37

        Retail = $2.34

4. XYZ Wholesaler sells bottles of liquid antacid to ABC Pharmacy for $2.86 per bottle. ABC Pharmacy retails the antacid for $4.95. This profit made on each bottle is $0.97. **Calculate the total markup and the overhead.**

Known Values

Wholesale = $2.86
Retail = $4.95
Profit = $0.97

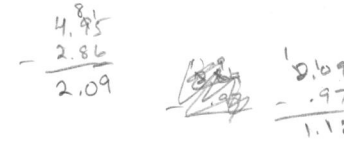

a) Calculate the markup using the following formula.

Markup = Retail - Wholesale

Markup = $4.95 - $2.86

Markup = $2.09

b) Calculate the overhead using the following formula.

Overhead = Markup - Profit

Overhead = $2.09 - $0.97

Overhead = $1.12

It is very important to be able to calculate the markup percentage. You should also be able to calculate the markup amount if given a markup percentage. Suppose a pharmacy needed to add a 15% markup to every product to cover overhead expenses and make a profit. A technician should be able to calculate the retail price using the 15% markup and the wholesale price. Carefully read through the following examples involving markup percentages.

**Note: "Markup" always refers to the dollar amount and "markup percentage" always refers to the percentage of the markup.

Rx Success™ Complete Guide to Medical Math

5. MNO Pharmacy must markup all items from XYZ Wholesaler by 15%. A bottle of 100 count metoprolol costs the pharmacy $9.85. **Calculate the markup and the retail price of the 100 count bottle.**

   Known Values

   Markup Percentage = 15%
   Wholesale = $9.85

   a) Calculate the markup using the following formula.

   $$\text{Markup} = \frac{\text{Markup Percentage} \times \text{Wholesale}}{100}$$

   $$\text{Markup} = \frac{15 \times \$9.85}{100}$$

   Markup = $1.48

   b) Calculate the retail price using the following formula.

   Retail = Wholesale + Markup

   Retail = $9.85 + $1.48

   Retail = $11.33

6. MNO Pharmacy sells a popular blood pressure cuff for the retail selling price of $18.75. The markup amount is $5.37. **Calculate the wholesale cost and the markup percentage for each cuff.**

   Known Values

   Retail = $18.75
   Markup = $5.37

Rx Success™ Complete Guide to Medical Math

    a) Calculate the wholesale cost using the following formula.

        Wholesale = Retail - Markup

        Wholesale = $18.75 - $5.37

        Wholesale = $13.38

    b) Calculate the markup percentage using the following formula.

$$\text{Markup Percentage} = \frac{\text{Markup}}{\text{Wholesale}} \times 100$$

$$\text{Markup Percentage} = \frac{\$5.37}{\$13.38} \times 100$$

        Markup Percentage = 40%

---

7. You can also determine the cost of individual prescriptions. For instance, suppose a 100 count bottle of naproxen sodium costs the pharmacy $35.72. **Calculate the wholesale cost of only 30 tablets.**

[Handwritten: $\frac{35.72}{100} = 0.36/\text{tablet} \times 30 = \$10.72$]

<u>Known Values</u>

Wholesale = $35.72 per 100 count bottle

    a) Calculate the wholesale price using the following formula.

$$\frac{100 \text{ tablets}}{\$35.72} = \frac{30 \text{ tablets}}{\$X}$$

        Note: We are using cross multiplication to solve this problem!

$$\frac{100 \text{ tablets}}{\$35.72} \diagdown\!\!\!\!\diagup \frac{30 \text{ tablets}}{\$X}$$

        100X = 1071.6

        Now, solve for X.

Rx Success™ Complete Guide to Medical Math

$$\frac{\cancel{100}X}{\cancel{100}} = \frac{1071.6}{100}$$

X = $10.72

---

8. The wholesale cost of a 500 count bottle of alprazolam is $84.17. A pharmacy sells a 30 count prescription for $21.50. **Calculate the markup and the markup percentage for a 30 count prescription.**

   Known Values

   Wholesale for 500 count = $84.17
   Retail for 30 count = $21.50

   (Handwritten work:
   $\frac{X}{30} = \frac{84.17}{500}$ 500X = 2525.10   X = 5.05

   21.50 − 5.05 = 16.45

   16.45 / 5.05 = 3.26 or 326%*)

   a) First, we must find the wholesale cost for 30 tablets. Calculate the wholesale price using the following formula.

   $$\frac{500 \text{ tablets}}{\$84.17} = \frac{30 \text{ tablets}}{\$X}$$

   $$\frac{500 \text{ tablets}}{\$84.17} \times \frac{30 \text{ tablets}}{\$X}$$

   500X = 2525.1

   Now, solve for X

   $$\frac{\cancel{500}X}{\cancel{500}} = \frac{2525.1}{500}$$

   X = $5.05

   b) Calculate the markup using the following formula.

   Markup = Retail − Wholesale

   Markup = $21.50 − $5.05

   Markup = $16.45

c) Calculate the markup percentage using the following formula.

$$\text{Markup Percentage} = \frac{\text{Markup}}{\text{Wholesale}} \times 100$$

$$\text{Markup Percentage} = \frac{\$16.45}{\$5.05} \times 100$$

Markup Percentage = 326%

Rx Success™ Complete Guide to Medical Math

Pharmaco-Economics – Tutor Sheets™

USE THIS WORKSHEET AS A GUIDE TO HELP YOU SOLVE THE HOMEWORK PROBLEMS!

1. The wholesale price on a box of 4X4 gauze pads is $1.78. The pharmacy markup is 32%. Calculate the retail price for two boxes of gauze pads.

   1.78 × 1.32 = 2.35
   2.35 × 2 = $4.70

Go to the formula sheet on page 251 and write the formulas you need below…

Formula #1
$$\text{Markup} = \frac{\text{Markup Percentage} \times \text{Wholesale}}{100}$$

Formula #2
$$\text{Retail} = \underline{\hspace{2in}} + \underline{\hspace{2in}}$$

Step One – Using formula #1, calculate the markup amount.

$\underline{\hspace{1in}}$ = $\underline{\hspace{0.75in}}$ X $\underline{\hspace{0.75in}}$ divided by 100
markup amount

Step Two – Using formula #2, and the markup amount, calculate the retail price.

$\underline{\hspace{1in}}$ = $\underline{\hspace{0.75in}}$ + $\underline{\hspace{0.75in}}$
retail price

Step Three – Remember, the problem asked for the price on **two** boxes of gauze pads. To find this price, simply multiply the retail price of one box, by two.

$\underline{\hspace{1.5in}}$ = $\underline{\hspace{0.75in}}$ X 2
retail price for 2 boxes   retail price

---

2. A pharmacy patient sells a bottle of 30-count over-the-counter histamine tablets for $18.50. The wholesale price was $12.34. By what percentage did the pharmacy markup this bottle of tablets?

Go to the formula sheet on page 251 and write the formulas you need below…

18.50 – 12.34 = 6.16 $\frac{6.16}{12.34} = 0.50$ or 50%

Rx Success™ Complete Guide to Medical Math

Formula #1

Markup = _____ - _____

Formula #2

Markup % = _____ X 100

Step One – Using formula #1, calculate the markup amount.

$_____ = _____ - _____
markup amount

Step Two – Using formula #2, and the markup amount, calculate the markup percentage.

_____ % = _____ X 100
markup %

---

3. Your pharmacy pays $287.03 for a 1000 count bottle of 100 mg atentolol tablets. The pharmacy adds a 27% markup and a $4.25 professional fee to every prescription. Calculate the retail price for a patient will the following prescription: Atenolol 100 mg. Take 1 tablet by mouth bid X 90 days.

   Step One – Calculate how many tablets the patient needs to fill the whole prescription by using cross multiplication.

   $$\frac{\text{tabs}}{1 \text{ day}} = \frac{\text{tabs}}{90 \text{ days}}$$

   Handwritten work:
   2 × 90 = 180

   $$\frac{\$x}{180} = \frac{\$287.03}{1000}$$

   1000x = 51665.40
   x = $51.67 is wholesale

   51.67 × 1.27 = 65.62 + 4.25 = $69.87

   Step Two – Calculate the wholesale price for the patient's prescription using cross multiplication and the wholesale price for the 1000 count bottle.

   $$\frac{1000 \text{ tabs}}{\$} = \frac{\text{tabs}}{\$ X}$$

Rx Success™ Complete Guide to Medical Math

Step Three – Using…
- The correct formula from the Formula Sheet
- The Wholesale Price from Step Two
- The Markup Percentage from the problem

Calculate the markup amount on the prescription.

$\$\underline{\hspace{2cm}}_{\text{markup amount}} = \underline{\hspace{2cm}} \times 100$

Step Four – Using…
- The correct formula from the Formula Sheet
- The Markup Amount from Step Three
- The Wholesale Price from Step Two

Calculate the retail price on the prescription.

$\$\underline{\hspace{2cm}}_{\text{retail price}} = \underline{\hspace{2cm}} + \underline{\hspace{2cm}}$

Step Four – Find the final price by adding the Pharmacy's Professional Fee to the retail price of the prescription.

$\$\underline{\hspace{2cm}}_{\text{final price}} = \underline{\hspace{2cm}}_{\text{retail price}} + \underline{\hspace{2cm}}_{\text{professional fee}}$

Answers to Tutor Sheets™ Calculations
1) $4.70   2) 50%   3) $69.87

Rx Success™ Complete Guide to Medical Math

Pharmaco-Economics - Homework

Use the previous sample problems and formula page to help you calculate the following problems. Round percents off to whole numbers and round dollar amounts to the nearest penny.

Solve the following Pharmaco-Economic Problems:

1. Wholesale = $5.16
   Markup = $0.85

   Retail = __6.01__   Markup Percentage = __16%__

2. Wholesale = $20.70
   Markup = $3.90

   Retail = __24.60__   Markup Percentage = __19%__

3. Wholesale = $12.73
   Markup = $6.47

   Retail = __19.20__   Markup Percentage = __51%__

4. Wholesale = $31.15
   Markup = $11.02

   Retail = __42.17__   Markup Percentage = __35%__

Rx Success™ Complete Guide to Medical Math

5. Wholesale = $9.58
   Markup = $5.90

   Retail = __15.48__   Markup Percentage = __62%__

6. Wholesale = $0.75
   Overhead = $2.90
   Profit = $0.90

   Retail = __4.55__   Markup Percentage = __507%__

7. Wholesale = $19.24
   Overhead = $6.12
   Profit = $5.12

   Retail = __30.48__   Markup Percentage = __58%__

8. Wholesale = $2.60
   Overhead = $1.05
   Profit = $0.82

   Retail = __4.47__   Markup Percentage = __72%__

Rx Success™ Complete Guide to Medical Math

9. Wholesale = $0.98
   Overhead = $1.23
   Profit = $1.58

   Retail = __3.79__   Markup Percentage = __287%__

10. Wholesale = $31.45
    Overhead = $8.76
    Profit = $9.17

    Retail = __49.38__   Markup Percentage = __57%__

11. Wholesale = $2.17
    Retail = $5.67

    Markup = __3.50__   Markup Percentage = __161%__

12. Wholesale = $17.01
    Retail = $72.34
    Overhead = $20.00

    Markup = __55.33__   Markup Percentage = __325%__   Profit = __35.33__

13. Retail = $4.80
    Wholesale = $0.76

    Markup = __4.04__   Markup Percentage = __532%__

Rx Success™ Complete Guide to Medical Math

14. Wholesale = $23.40
    Markup Percentage = 32%

    Retail = __30.89__   Markup = __7.49__

15. Markup Percentage = 12.5%
    Wholesale = $6.81

    Retail = __7.66__   Markup = __0.85__

16. Wholesale = $3.92
    Markup Percentage = 110%

    Retail = __8.23__   Markup = __4.31__

17. Markup Percentage = 78%
    Wholesale = $0.49

    Retail = __$0.87__   Markup = __0.38__

18. Retail = $109.05
    Wholesale = $42.80

    Markup = __66.+5__   Markup Percentage = __155%__

Rx Success™ Complete Guide to Medical Math

19. Retail = $35.21
    Wholesale = $17.32

    Markup = ____17.89____   Markup Percentage = ____103%____

20. Retail = $74.99
    Wholesale = $30.20

    Markup = ____44.79____   Markup Percentage = ____148%____

21. The wholesale price on a bottle of aspirin is $0.85. The pharmacy markup is 37%. Calculate the retail price for a bottle of aspirin.

    Retail = ____1.16____

22. The wholesale price on a blood pressure cuff is $24.90. Calculate the retail price after adding a 25% markup.

    Retail = ____31.13____

23. The pharmacy pays $9.17 for a 60 count bottle of famotidine tablets. After marking the bottle up by 115%, what is the final retail price for this bottle?

    Retail = ____19.72____

Rx Success™ Complete Guide to Medical Math

24. A pharmacy buys a 100 count bottle of OTC antihistamine for $2.70 and marks it up by 53%. How much would a consumer pay for the entire bottle?

Retail = __4.13__

25. A consumer pays $4.60 for a four-ounce bottle of guaifenesin. The wholesale price was $3.70. Calculate the markup amount. Calculate the percent markup.

Markup = __0.90__   Markup Percentage = __24%__

26. A pharmacy customer buys a bottle of 50 count blood glucose test strips for $45.80. The wholesale price was $28.38. By what percentage did the pharmacy markup this bottle of test strips?

Markup Percentage = __61%__

27. If a pharmacy customer pays $13.53 for an over-the-counter item and the pharmacy wholesale price was $10.80, calculate the markup percentage on this item.

Markup Percentage = __25%__

28. Calculate the markup percentage on a bottle of chlorpheniramine. The retail price is $5.90 and the wholesale price was $2.15.

Markup Percentage = __174%__

Rx Success™ Complete Guide to Medical Math

29. The wholesale price on 45 tablets of a prescription medication is $0.92. Calculate the patient price if the pharmacy markup is 15% and the professional fee is $9.50

Retail = __10.56__

30. The wholesale price on 30 amoxicillin capsules is $3.15. Calculate the retail price if the pharmacy adds a 23% markup to every prescription and a professional fee of $3.25.

Retail = __7.12__

31. A patient needs to fill a prescription for 90 tablets of metoprolol. The wholesale price is $8.70. Calculate the retail price if the pharmacy adds a 17% markup and a $4.25 professional fee to every prescription.

Retail = __14.43__

32. A pharmacy can purchase a 500 count bottle of acetaminophen/hydrocodone for a wholesale price of $134.75. The pharmacy adds a 20% markup and a $4.80 professional fee to every prescription. Calculate the retail price for a prescription with the following directions: Take 1-2 tablets by mouth every 4 to 6 hours as needed for pain. Disp: #30

$$\frac{\$x}{30} = \frac{\$134.75}{500}$$

$500x = 4042.50$

$x = \$8.09$ wholesale for 30 tabs

Retail = __14.51__

33. The wholesale price on a 100 count bottle of a prescription antacid is $82.10. The pharmacy marks everything up by 15% and adds a $5.60 professional fee to every prescription. A patient presents a prescription with the following directions: Take 2 tablets by mouth every 4 hours for seven days. Calculate the retail price for this prescription.

84 tabs

$$\frac{\$x}{84} = \frac{\$82.10}{100}$$
$$100x = 6896.40$$
$$x = 68.96$$

Retail = __84.91__

34. A pharmacy pays $123.09 for 500 tablets of a drug. The pharmacy marks everything up by 12% and charges an $8.25 professional fee on every prescription. Calculate the price on a prescription for 30 tablets of this drug.

$$\frac{\$x}{30} = \frac{\$123.09}{500}$$
$$500x = 3692.70$$
$$x = 7.39$$

Retail = __16.52__

35. A pharmacy can purchase 100 count bottles of a prescription antidepressant for $37.09 each. How much money does the pharmacy save by buying a 500 count bottle of the same medication for $117.30?

37.09 × 5 = 185.45 − 117.30 = 68.15

$ __68.15__

36. A pharmacy cost on one tablet of a very expensive antibiotic is $1.07. The pharmacy adds a $7.15 professional fee and a 30% markup to every prescription. Calculate the retail price on the following prescription for this antibiotic: Take 2 tablets on day one. Then take one tablet daily for the next four days.

6 tabs × 1.07 = 6.42

Retail = __15.50__

37. The pharmacy is able to purchase a 1000-tablet bottle of a drug for $230.95, while 50 count bottles of the same medication cost $23.15. Calculate the total pharmacy savings by buying one bulk container of 1000 tabs.

    20 × 23.15 = 463.00 − 230.95 = 232.05

    $ __232.05__

38. A pharmacy can purchase 30 count bottles of an antibiotic for $8.68 each. It can purchase 100 count bottles for $22.80 each. What is the total amount that the pharmacy can save by buying three, 100 count bottles of this antibiotic?

    300 tab total
    3 × 22.80 = 68.40   10 × 8.68 = 86.80 − 68.40 = 18.40

    $ __18.40__

39. A pharmacy can purchase 100 count bottles of metronidazole for $34.00 each. The cost of a 500 count bottle is $135.32. How much money would the pharmacy save on 1000 tablets by buying the 500 count bottles?

    2 × 135.32 = 270.64
    10 × 34 = 340 − 270.64 = 69.36

    $ __69.36__

40. If a pharmacy buys a box of bandages for $2.27 and the markup is $1.42, calculate the retail price and the percent markup for the gauze pads?

    Retail = __3.69__   Markup Percentage = __63%__

41. The wholesale price on ketone testing strips is $10.53 for 50 count. The overhead for the item is $3.15 and the pharmacy would like to make $5.78 profit. What is the retail price?

    Retail = __19.46__

Rx Success™ Complete Guide to Medical Math

42. Your pharmacy orders a case of liquid nutritional supplement for a customer at a cost of $16.29. Your pharmacy will sell the case for $34.80. If the overhead on the case is $11.63, what is the pharmacy's profit?

$$34.80 - 16.29 = 18.51 - 11.63 =$$

Profit = __6.88__

43. Bob's Pharmacy is selling a package of throat lozenges for $2.17. You know that the overhead is $0.54 and the pharmacy is making $0.63 per package. What is the wholesale price of the cough drops?

Wholesale = __$1.00__

44. A pharmacy charges a 22% markup and a $4.65 professional fee on every prescription. If the pharmacy pays $7.50 for an item, what is the retail price of that item?

Retail = __13.80__

45. A pharmacy buys 500 tablets of a prescription antihistamine for $185.00. The pharmacy adds a 9% markup and a $5.95 professional fee to every prescription. What is the total retail price for a bottle of 500 tablets? How much would the pharmacy charge to fill a prescription for 30 tablets?

Retail for 500 tabs = __207.60__   Retail for 30 tabs = __18.05__

$$\frac{\$x}{30} = \frac{\$185.00}{500}$$

$$500x = 5550$$

$$x = 11.10 \text{ wholesale}$$

Page - 292

46. A pharmacy's cost on one tablet of a very expensive antibiotic is $2.09. The pharmacy adds a 12% markup and a $7.25 professional fee to every prescription. How much would a patient pay to fill a prescription for seven tablets of this antibiotic?

7 x 2.09 = 14.63

Retail = 23.64

Rx Success™ Complete Guide to Medical Math

Chapter Sixteen

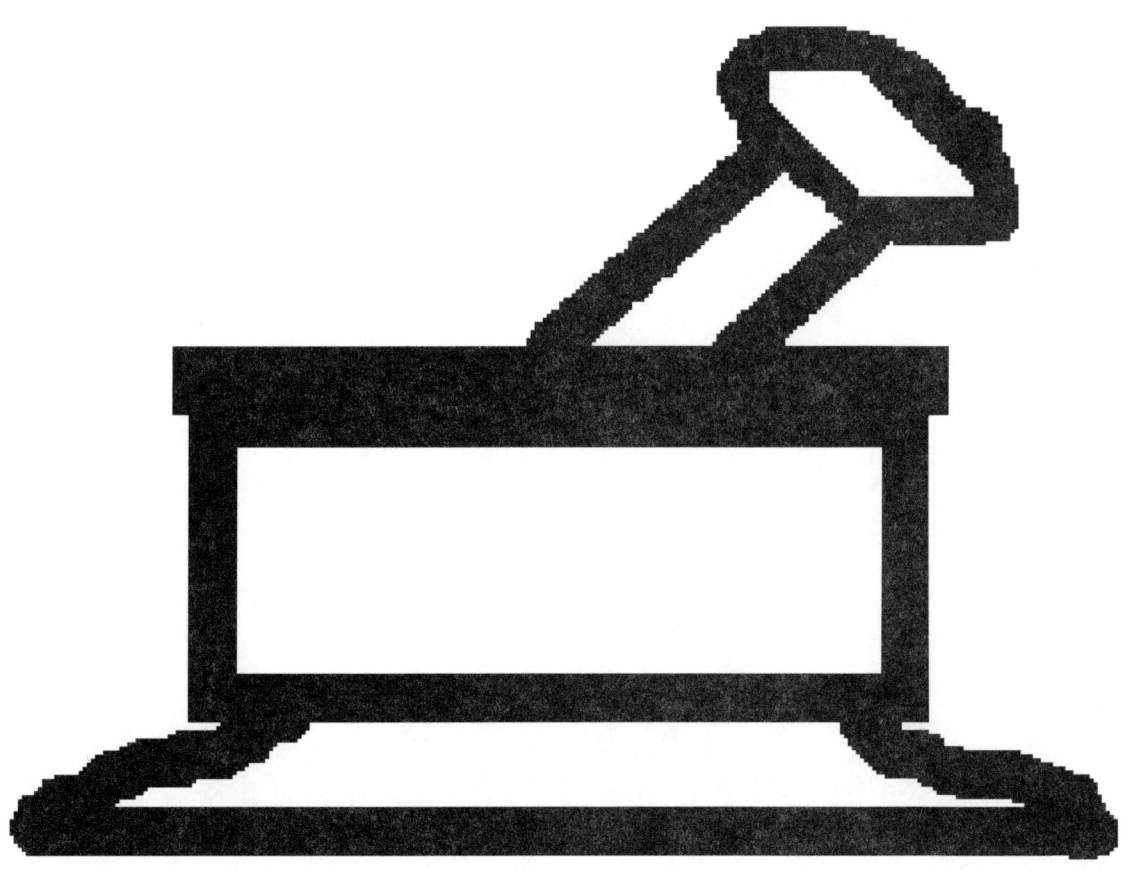

Homework Answer Key

Rx Success™ Complete Guide to Medical Math

Homework Answer Key

Conversion Factor Worksheet
Fill in the correct conversion "codes" for the equivalents (page 15).

1. 2.2 lb
2. 30 ml
3. 15 ml
4. 60 mg
5. 1 qt
6. 480 ml
7. 5 ml
8. 16 oz
9. 2 pt
10. 454 g

Roman Numeral Conversions – Homework
Write the Roman Numeral equivalents for the following numbers (page 27).

1. IV
2. X
3. XVIII
4. XXIII
5. IX
6. XIV
7. XI
8. XXVII
9. XIX
10. XXX
11. LIV
12. XXV
13. XVI
14. XLV
15. L
16. XXXII
17. CI
18. CIX
19. LXXV
20. LXXXIV
21. XCIII
22. CCLXXV
23. CLIII
24. CD
25. CCCXXIII
26. CDL
27. DI
28. LXXXVII
29. DCXV
30. CCXXXI
31. DCCCLXX
32. D
33. DCCXC
34. CDXXV
35. MCCL
36. DCCLXIV
37. CXXIII
38. MD
39. MM
40. MMIII

Write the Roman Numeral equivalents for the following numbers (page 29).

1. 7
2. 3
3. 9
4. 11
5. 110
6. 1900
7. 40
8. 60
9. 400
10. 617
11. 84
12. 2003
13. 1972

Rx Success™ Complete Guide to Medical Math

14. 57
15. 123
16. 19
17. 600
18. 94
19. 186
20. 999

Military/Standard Time – Homework
Convert the following Standard Times to Military (page 37).

1. 0100 hours
2. 0200 hours
3. 0300 hours
4. 0400 hours
5. 0500 hours
6. 0600 hours
7. 0700 hours
8. 0800 hours
9. 0900 hours
10. 1000 hours
11. 1100 hours
12. 1200 hours
13. 1300 hours
14. 1400 hours
15. 1500 hours
16. 1600 hours
17. 1700 hours
18. 1800 hours
19. 1900 hours
20. 2000 hours
21. 2100 hours
22. 2200 hours
23. 2300 hours
24. 2400 hours
25. 0131 hours
26. 1217 hours
27. 2030 hours
28. 1523 hours
29. 0918 hours
30. 1310 hours
31. 0830 hours
32. 1955 hours
33. 0315 hours
34. 0745 hours
35. 2232 hours
36. 1157 hours
37. 2320 hours
38. 1830 hours
39. 1745 hours
40. 1430 hours

Convert the following Military Times to Standard (page 38).

1. 12:00 noon
2. 1:00 pm
3. 2:00 pm
4. 3:00 pm
5. 4:00 pm
6. 5:00 pm
7. 6:00 pm
8. 7:00 pm
9. 8:00 pm
10. 9:00 pm
11. 10:00 pm
12. 11:00 pm
13. 12:00 midnight
14. 1:00 am
15. 2:00 am
16. 3:00 am
17. 4:00 am
18. 5:00 am
19. 6:00 am
20. 7:00 am
21. 8:00 am
22. 9:00 am
23. 10:00 am
24. 11:00 am
25. 12:01 am
26. 4:25 pm
27. 3:15 am
28. 10:45 pm
29. 8:30 pm
30. 11:56 am
31. 12:01 pm
32. 7:25 pm
33. 7:45 am
34. 9:02 am
35. 12:50 pm
36. 9:45 pm
37. 11:18 pm
38. 6:20 am
39. 5:45 pm
40. 2:30 pm

Rx Success™ Complete Guide to Medical Math

Temperature Conversions – Homework
Convert the following temperatures to C° or F° (page 49).

1. 87.8° F
2. 48.4° C
3. -8.8° C
4. 212° F
5. 22° C
6. 192°.2 F
7. 62.6° F
8. 37.4° C
9. 0° C
10. -17.6° C
11. 74.3° F
12. -24.2° C
13. 5° F
14. 209.3° F
15. 35.8° C
16. 36.6° C
17. 35.6° F
18. -9.9° C
19. 46.4° F
20. 104° F
21. 86° F
22. 15.4° C
23. 99° C
24. 29.7° C
25. 59° F
26. -58° F
27. 39.6° C
28. 32° F
29. -19.8° C
30. -4° F

Metric Conversions – Homework
Metric Measure of Dry Weight – Fill in the metric equivalents for the given weight values (page 59).

	mcg	mg	g	kg
1.	815,500	**815.5**	0.8155	0.0008155
2.	750,000	**750**	0.75	0.00075
3.	**82.3**	0.0823	0.0000823	0.0000000823
4.	4500	4.5	**0.0045**	0.0000045
5.	1,120,000,000	1,120,000	1120	**1.12**
6.	750	**0.75**	0.00075	0.00000075
7.	45,000,000	45,000	**45**	0.045
8.	250,000	250	0.25	**0.00025**
9.	125,000	**125**	0.125	0.000125
10.	75	**0.075**	0.000075	0.000000075
11.	105,000,000	105,000	**105**	0.105
12.	1,007,500,000	1,007,500	1007.5	**1.0075**
13.	10,200,000,000	10,200,000	10,200	**10.2**
14.	10,000,000	**10,000**	10	0.01
15.	950,000,000	950,000	**950**	0.95

Metric Measure of Volume – Fill in the metric equivalents for the given liquid volume values (page 59).

	mcl	ml	L	kl
1.	62,500	**62.5**	0.0625	0.0000625
2.	70,000	**70**	0.07	0.00007
3.	190,000	**190**	0.19	0.00019
4.	1,200,000	1200	**1.2**	0.0012
5.	31,050	**31.05**	0.03105	0.00003105
6.	75	**0.075**	0.000075	0.000000075
7.	8,750,000	8750	8.75	**0.00875**
8.	150,000	150	0.15	**0.00015**
9.	7,024,000	7024	**7.024**	0.007024

Rx Success™ Complete Guide to Medical Math

	mcl	ml	L	kl
10.	2050	2.05	**0.00205**	0.00000205
11.	10,000,000	10,000	**10**	0.01
12.	208,000,000	208,000	208	**0.208**
13.	1,000,000,000	1,000,000	1000	**1**
14.	8000.5	**8.0005**	0.0080005	0.0000080005
15.	2,030,000	2030	**2.03**	0.00203

Metric Measure of Length – Fill in the metric equivalents for the given length values (page 60).

	mcm	mm	m	km
1.	700,000	700	**0.7**	0.0007
2.	8500	8.5	0.0085	**0.0000085**
3.	**115,000**	115	0.115	0.000115
4.	1250	1.25	**0.00125**	0.00000125
5.	1,120,000,000	1,120,000	1120	**1.12**
6.	815	**0.815**	0.000815	0.000000815
7.	9,100,000	9100	**9.1**	0.0091
8.	250,000	250	0.25	**0.00025**
9.	6,050,000,000	6,050,000	6050	**6.05**
10.	**900**	0.9	0.0009	0.0000009
11.	7,000,000	7000	**7**	0.007
12.	10,205,000	10,205	10.205	**0.010205**
13.	4,000,000	4,000	4	**0.004**
14.	127,500,000	**127,500**	127.5	0.1275
15.	425,000	**425**	0.425	0.000425

<u>Fraction/Decimal/Ratio/Percent Conversions – Homework</u>
Fill in the following table of equivalent measurements. Reduce to lowest terms where appropriate (page 71).

	Percent	Ratio	Fraction	Decimal
1.	0.01%	1:10,000	1/10,000	**0.0001**
2.	20%	**1:5**	1/5	0.2
3.	3.1%	1:32	**3/96**	0.031
4.	17.5%	7:40	7/40	**0.175**
5.	40%	2:5	2/5	**0.4**
6.	0.8%	1:125	1/125	**0.008**
7.	**15%**	3:20	3/20	0.15
8.	13.3%	2:15	**2/15**	0.133
9.	62.5%	5:8	5/8	**0.625**
10.	8.3%	1:12	**1/12**	0.083
11.	1%	**1:100**	1/100	0.01
12.	**1.25%**	1:80	1/80	0.0125
13.	14.3%	3:21	**15/105**	0.143
14.	50%	1:2	**1.5/3**	0.5
15.	1.7%	**3:180**	1/60	0.017

Rx Success™ Complete Guide to Medical Math

Percent	Ratio	Fraction	Decimal
16. 0.19%	**1.75:900**	7/3600	0.0019
17. 0.5%	1:200	1/200	**0.005**
18. 49.5%	50:101	**7/14.14**	0.495
19. **0.0025%**	1:40,000	1/40,000	0.000025
20. **0.08%**	1:1250	1/1250	0.0008
21. **875%**	35:4	35/4	8.75
22. 0.033%	**1:3000**	1/3000	0.00033
23. 15.3%	**115:750**	23/150	0.153
24. 9%	9:100	**9/100**	0.09
25. 25%	1:4	**2.5/10**	0.25
26. 0.8%	1:125	1/125	**0.008**
27. 1%	1:100	1/100	**0.01**
28. **11.5%**	23:200	23/200	0.115
29. 4.98%	**7.5:150.5**	15/301	0.0498
30. 35%	7:20	7/20	**0.35**
31. 1.5%	3:200	3/200	**0.015**
32. **12.6%**	63:500	63/500	0.126
33. 0.1%	1:1000	**10.1/10100**	0.001
34. 2000%	**1:0.05**	20/1	20
35. 1000%	10:1	**250/25**	10
36. 6%	3:50	3/50	**0.06**
37. **90%**	9:10	9/10	0.9
38. **0.225%**	9:4000	9/4000	0.00225
39. 1.7%	**1.5:90**	1/60	0.017
40. 4%	**2:50**	1/25	0.04
41. 80%	4:5	**4/5**	0.8
42. 10.5%	21:200	21/200	**0.105**
43. 400%	4:1	**12.5/3.125**	4
44. 2000%	**100:5**	20/1	20
45. **8.75%**	7:80	7/80	0.0875
46. 10%	1:10	**1,000/10,000**	0.1
47. 0.025%	1:4000	**50/200,000**	0.00025
48. 0.001%	1:100,000	1/100,000	**0.00001**
49. **10.1%**	101:1000	101/1000	0.101
50. 8.8%	**12:136**	3/34	0.088

Cross Multiplication – Homework
Use cross multiplication to calculate the following problems (page 87).

1. 1500 sec
2. 6960 sec
3. 151.2 in
4. 9 in
5. 510 min
6. 1.5 ft

7. 6 min
8. 1 hr
9. 1.2 min
10. 52 yd
11. 20 min
12. 50 ft
13. 2,000 yd
14. 3.1 min
15. 30.5 yd
16. 2916 in
17. 5.94 yd
18. 2.28 hr
19. 334.8 in
20. 61,200 sec

Apothecary, Household and Metric Conversions – Homework
Use cross multiplication to calculate the following problems (page 103).

1. 32 pt
2. 12 gr
3. 20 t
4. 97.5 ml
5. 28 dr
6. 936 mg
7. 82.5 ml
8. 0.75 gr
9. 402 ml
10. 450 mg
11. 60 dr
12. 0.125 dr
13. 105 ml
14. 450 ml
15. 28 oz
16. 31.25 gr
17. 320 ml
18. 3600 ml
19. 4 pt
20. 2.4 qt

The following problems involve 2-step conversions (page 105)

21. 432 oz
22. 0.45 g
23. 2520 dr
24. 2 oz
25. 0.25 oz
26. 18.75 dr
27. 2.29 pt
28. 6 pt
29. 48 t
30. 1 T
31. 8 oz
32. 2.69 pt
33. 2500 gr
34. 420 mg
35. 390 dr
36. 1.28 pt

Rx Success™ Complete Guide to Medical Math

37. 100.8 t
38. 1.25 pt
39. 48 oz
40. 1.25 gr
41. 1080 mg
42. 240 ml
43. 33.6 T
44. 16.88 qt
45. 345.6 t

Dosage Calculations Step One – Homework
Using fractions and cross multiplication, calculate the following doses (page 119).

1. 7.5 ml
2. 1 ml
3. 0.75 ml
4. 2.25 ml
5. 3.75 ml
6. 1.4 ml
7. 0.75 ml
8. 40 ml
9. 0.25 ml
10. 200 ml
11. 800 mg
12. 0.32 mg
13. 1.6 ml
14. 100 mEq
15. 25 mg
16. 6.88 ml
17. 72 mg
18. NO, 8 ml
19. YES
20. 3 ml
21. NO, 1.2 ml
22. 2.25 ml
23. 4.38 ml
24. 0.53 mg
25. 100 mEq
26. 15 ml
27. 2.5 ml
28. NO, 0.6 ml
29. NO, 4.5 ml
30. 70 ml
31. 1500 ml
32. 224 ml
33. 3937.5 mg
34. 4.5 mg
35. 600 mg

Rx Success™ Complete Guide to Medical Math

Dosage Calculations Step Two – Homework
Calculate the following body weight equivalents (page 139).

1. **Pounds to Kilograms**
    a) 21.82 kg
    b) 50.91 kg
    c) 6.36 kg
    d) 16.14 kg
    e) 100 kg
    f) 4.77 kg
    g) 45.45 kg
    h) 22.77 kg
    i) 10.45 kg
    j) 46.82 kg
    k) 1 kg
    l) 13.64 kg
    m) 8.18 kg
    n) 80.91 kg
    o) 76.59 kg

2. **Kilograms to Pounds**
    a) 220 lb
    b) 34.1 lb
    c) 19.8 lb
    d) 154 lb
    e) 264 lb
    f) 118.8 lb
    g) 51.7 lb
    h) 176 lb
    i) 99 lb
    j) 57.64 lb
    k) 68.2 lb
    l) 209 lb
    m) 169.4 lb
    n) 180.4 lb
    o) 83.6 lb

Calculate the doses for the patients in the following problems (page 140).

3. 84 mg
4. 1125 mg
5. 374 mg
6. 2.1 mg
7. 18 mg
8. 1443.18 mg
9. 0.41 mg
10. 709.09 mg
11. 13.64 mg
12. 1227.3 mg
13. 20.45 mg
14. 310.92 mg
15. 118.18 mg
16. 143.17 mg
17. 5112.5 kg
18. 528.41 mg
19. 300 mg
20. 14,400 mg
21. 1610 mg

22. 125 mg
23. 92.26 mg
24. 0.82 mg
25. 31.37 mg
26. 0.39 mg
27. 625 mg
28. 6.48 mg
29. 37,500 mg
30. YES
31. NO
32. 0.84 ml
33. 0.17 ml
34. 17.05 ml
35. 3.15 ml
36. 0.74 ml
37. 2.24 ml
38. 2.05 ml
39. 1.77 ml
40. NO
41. YES
42. NO

Insulin Calculations – Homework (page 163)
a) Calculate the following insulin doses.
b) Indicate what size insulin syringe will be used.

1. a) 0.26 ml   b) 1/3 cc
2. a) 0.75 ml   b) 1 cc
3. a) 0.14 ml   b) 1/3 cc
4. a) 0.3 ml   b) 1/3 cc
5. a) 0.07 ml   b) 1/3 cc
6. a) 0.9 ml   b) 1 cc
7. a) 0.54 ml   b) 1 cc
8. a) 0.17 ml   b) 1/3 cc
9. a) 0.34 ml   b) 1/2 cc
10. a) 0.83 ml   b) 1 cc

11. 60 U
12. 1.2 ml
13. 15 U
14. 4.2 ml
15. 0.32 ml
16. 0.75 ml
17. 0.48 ml
18. a) Regular   b) 0.87 ml   c) 1 cc
19. a) Regular   b) 0.67 ml   c) 1 cc
20. a) Regular   b) 0.74 ml   c) 1 cc
21. a) Regular   b) 0.85 ml   c) 1 cc
22. 0.62 ml
23. 0.45 ml
24. YES
25. a) Regular   b) 0.25 ml   c) 0.7 ml   d) 1 cc

Rx Success™ Complete Guide to Medical Math

Percent Solutions – Homework
Calculate the following problems using the percents given (page 183).

1. 3 g
2. 11.25 g
3. 7.5 g
4. 5.63 g
5. 150 g
6. 595 g
7. 2.5 g
8. 1.13 g
9. 1.58 g
10. 1.88 g
11. 6000 ml
12. 544.8 g
13. 33 full bottles
14. 3%
15. 5%
16. 2.5%
17. 15 g
18. 5%
19. 10,896 g
20. 10%
21. 2%
22. 0.03%
23. 0.025%
24. 0.5%

IV Drip Rate Calculations – Homework
Calculate the following IV drip rates (page 211).

1. 150 ml/hr
2. 250 ml/hr
3. 1.25 ml/min
4. 3.33 ml/min; 33 gtts/min
5. 1.67 ml/min; 100 gtts/min
6. 56 gtts/min
7. 4.17 ml/min; 50 gtts/min
8. 0.83 ml/min; 25 gtts/min
9. 1.39 ml/min; 14 gtts/min
10. 3.33 ml/min; 50 gtts/min
11. 4.17 ml/min; 83 gtts/min
12. 2.08 ml/min; 125 gtts/min
13. 2.5 ml/min; 30 gtts/min
14. 1.67 ml/min; 25 gtts/min
15. 54 gtts/min
16. 0.83 ml/min; 50 gtts/min
17. 1.88 ml/min; 28 gtts/min
18. 0.5 ml/min; 5 gtts/min
19. 3.33 ml/min; 33 gtts/min
20. 4.17 ml/min; 250 gtts/min

Rx Success™ Complete Guide to Medical Math

Calculate the following total infusion times from the information given (page 216).

1. 233.33 min
2. 150 min
3. 30 min
4. 83.33 min
5. 62.5 min
6. 62.5 min
7. 566.67 min
8. 384.62 min
9. 500 min
10. 64.26 min
11. 50 min
12. 142.86 min
13. 113.33 min
14. 233.33 min
15. 300 min
16. 120 min
17. 200 min
18. 77.78 min
19. 171.43 min
20. 100 min

In the following problems, solve for the amount of drug given per unit of time (page 219).

1. 0.42 mg/min
2. 0.17 mEq/min
3. 8.33 mg/min
4. 0.21 U/min
5. 6.67 mg/min
6. 140 mg
7. 90 mg
8. 312.5 ml

Solve the following Advanced Drip Rate Calculations (page 221).

1. 0.11 mEq/min
2. 4.17 mg/min
3. 2.22 mg/min
4. 10 gtts/min
5. 31.25 U/min; 800 min
6. 1.33 mEq/min
7. 42 gtts/min; 11.11 mg/min
8. 236.59 min; 6.34 mg/min
9. 142.86 min; 4.2 mg/min
10. 23 gtts/min; 150.21 min
11. 50 gtts/min; 0.21 U/min
12. 50 gtts/min; 5 mg/min
13. 427.35 min; 0.59 mg/min
14. 120 gtts/min
15. 775 mg; 688.89 min
16. 15 gtts/min; 250 min
17. 0.09 U/min; 55.2 U; 640 min
18. 649 min; 9 gtts/min

Rx Success™ Complete Guide to Medical Math

Alligations - Homework (page 241)
a) **Calculate the ratio needed.**
b) **Calculate the amount needed for each solution.**

1.   a) 1:3
        b) 37.5 ml of 10%; 112.5 ml of 2%

2.   a) 7:6
        b) 377 ml of 70%; 323 ml of 5%

3.   a) 1:1
        b) 12.5 ml of 15%; 12.5 ml of 11%

4.   a) 2:3
        b) 600 ml of 9%; 900 ml of 1.5%

5.   a) 7:9 (3.5:4.5 is fine also)
        b) 1225 ml of 10%; 1575 ml of 2%

6.   a) 1:2
        b) 433 ml of 5%; 867 ml of 2%

7.   a) 5:23 (12.5:57.5 is fine also)
        b) 134 ml of 70%; 616 ml of distilled water

8.   a) 1:13
        b) 6 ml of 70%; 74 ml of distilled water

9.   a) 6:19 (1.2:3.8 is fine also)
        b) 36 ml of 5%; 114 ml of distilled water

10.   a) 11:16 (0.275:0.4 is fine also)
        b) 20 ml of 0.9%; 30 ml of 0.225%

11.   280 ml of 25%; 350 ml of 7%
12.   612.5 ml of 3%
13.   4 bottles
14.   28 ml of 4%; 47 ml of distilled water
15.   770 ml of 70%; 1730 ml of 5%
16.   14 ml of 80%
17.   819 ml of 70%; 3681 ml of 15%
18.   12.5 ml of 0.5%; 112.5 ml of alcohol
19.   429 ml of 70%; 171 ml saline solution
20.   20 ml of 10%; 60 ml of dextrose solution
21.   3.6 g of 5% ointment; 356.4 g of Aquaphor
22.   170 g of 1%; 511 g of Eucerin
23.   500 ml of sterile water
24.   320 ml of distilled water
25.   743 ml of normal saline

Rx Success™ Complete Guide to Medical Math

Pediatric Dosage Calculations – Homework
Follow the instructions to calculate the following pediatric dosages using the formulas from the previous section (page 257).

1. 392 mg
2. 48 mg
3. 42 mg
4. 25 mg
5. 75 mg
6. 40 mg
7. 4.67 mg
8. 83.33 mg
9. 102.27 mg
10. 319 mg
11. 6,000 U
12. 36.67 mg
13. 2 gr
14. 156.25 mg
15. 330 mg
16. 0.07 mg
17. 0.008 mg
18. 19.42 mg
19. 353.76 mg
20. 173.41 mg
21. 59 mg
22. 124.28 mg
23. 104.05 mg
24. 711 mg
25. 83.24 mg
26. 33.24 mg
27. Yes
28. No, the child's ordered dose does not exceed the daily limit.
29. Yes, the child's ordered dose exceeds the daily limit.
30. No, the ordered dose is not safe.
31. Yes, the ordered dose is appropriate.
32. No, the order is not appropriate.
33. Yes, the dose it correct.
34. Yes, the child's dose exceeds the maximum limit.
35. No, the dose does not exceed the maximum limit.
36. No, the dose does not exceed the recommendations.
37. No, the dose does not exceed the recommendations.
38. Between 153.18 mg and 229.77 mg per day

Pharmaco-Economics – Homework
Calculate the following Pharmaco-Economic Problems (page 283).

1. Retail: $6.01   Markup Percentage: 16%
2. Retail: $24.60   Markup Percentage: 19%
3. Retail: $19.20   Markup Percentage: 51%
4. Retail: $42.17   Markup Percentage: 35%
5. Retail: $15.48   Markup Percentage: 62%
6. Retail: $4.55   Markup Percentage: 507%
7. Retail: $30.48   Markup Percentage: 58%
8. Retail: $4.47   Markup Percentage: 72%
9. Retail: $3.79   Markup Percentage: 287%
10. Retail: $49.38 Markup Percentage: 57%

11. Markup: $3.50   Markup Percentage: 161%
12. Markup: $55.33   Markup Percentage: 325%   Profit: $35.33
13. Markup: $4.04   Markup Percentage: 532%
14. Retail: $30.89   Markup: $7.49
15. Retail: $7.66   Markup: $0.85
16. Retail: $8.23   Markup: $4.31
17. Retail: $0.87   Markup: $0.38
18. Markup: $66.25   Markup Percentage: 155%
19. Markup: $17.89   Markup Percentage: 103%
20. Markup: $44.79   Markup Percentage: 148%
21. Retail: $1.16
22. Retail: $31.12
23. Retail: $19.72
24. Retail: $4.13
25. Markup: $0.90   Markup Percentage: 24%
26. Markup Percentage: 61%
27. Markup Percentage: 25%
28. Markup Percentage: 174%
29. Retail: $10.56
30. Retail: $7.12
31. Retail: $14.43
32. Retail: $14.50
33. Retail: $84.91
34. Retail: $16.52
35. $68.15
36. Retail: $15.50
37. $232.05
38. $18.40
39. $69.36
40. Retail: $3.69   Markup Percentage: 63%
41. Retail: $19.46
42. Profit: $6.88
43. Wholesale: $1.00
44. Retail: $13.80
45. Retail for 500 tabs: $207.60   Retail for 30 tabs: $18.05
46. Retail: $23.64

Notes

Notes

Notes

Notes

Notes

Notes

Rx Success™ Complete Guide to Medical Math

Product Catalog/Order Form

Come Visit us at www.rxtechsuccess.com

To order *Rx Success™* Products On-Line

Or...

Use the *Rx Success™* Order Form that follows!

Or...

Call Us Toll-Free at (866) 898-9374

Rx Success™
Compounding Kit - $249.95
Have you always wanted to learn more about Extemporaneous Compounding? Would you like to practice these skills at home? Earn your Compounding Certificate and 12 CE credits with the *Rx Success™* Compounding Kit!

When you purchase this kit, you will receive everything you need to safely practice your extemporaneous compounding at home! You will receive:
- *Rx Success™* Compounding – Techniques and Theory for the Pharmacy Technician – This manual is written specifically for Pharmacy Technicians! You will find detailed, easy-to-understand explanations of compounding techniques *and* an extensive section on compounding math!
- *Rx Success™* Workbook – Your workbook contains practice recipes, compounding logs and quizzes that may be returned to an *Rx Success™* Instructor for grading.
- Mortar and Pestle
- Counting Tray
- Compounding Spatula
- Ingredients
- Recipes for Practice Formulations

When successfully completed, you will receive a Compounding Certificate and 12 hours of Continuing Education credit for your work!

You can also order this upgrade on-line at www.rxtechsuccess.com

Rx Success™ Complete Guide to Medical Math

Rx Success™
National Certification Review Manual - $39.95

Are you or someone you know studying to pass the Pharmacy Technician National Certification Exam? Get the very best study tool available and order the *Rx Success*™ National Certification Review Manual!

You can place your order by calling our toll-free number (866) 898-9374 or order on-line at www.rxtechsuccess.com

The 9th Edition of the original *Rx Success*™ Manual contains over 440 pages of essential information!

Don't Be Caught Without This Book! Get the *Rx Success*™ Advantage Today!

Rx Success™
Exam Prep Phlash™ Cards - $19.95
Looking for a portable, fun way to study for the National Certification Exam?

Rx Success™ Exam Prep Phlash™ Cards are the answer! Each card presents a question with four multiple choice answers. On the back, the correct answer is listed with a detailed explanation. Let friends or family members help you prepare with these easy-to-use cards! You can also order these cards on-line at www.rxtechsuccess.com

---

Rx Success™
Drug Memorization Phlash™ Cards - $25.95
Need help memorizing all those medications?

Our *Rx Success*™ Drug Memorization Phlash™ Cards can help you with the difficult task of drug memorization AND pronunciation! These 250 drug cards are portable, easily taken *anywhere* so you can study *anytime*! Flipping through these cards helps you learn the brand with generic equivalents (complete with pronunciations), indications and classifications, dosage forms and availability and DEA schedules! You can also order these cards on-line at www.rxtechsuccess.com

We can help you learn the information *YOU NEED TO KNOW*!

Extra! Extra!

Sign up today for a *free* subscription of this quarterly E-Newsletter!
Every quarter, you will receive a copy of

The Rx Philes™

Go to www.rxtechsuccess.com and click on the "Free Newsletter" icon!

Rx Success™ Complete Guide to Medical Math

Don't forget to visit www.rxtechsuccess.com often to check out the latest wisdom from Tess Perle – Technician Extraordinaire!

Tess Perle

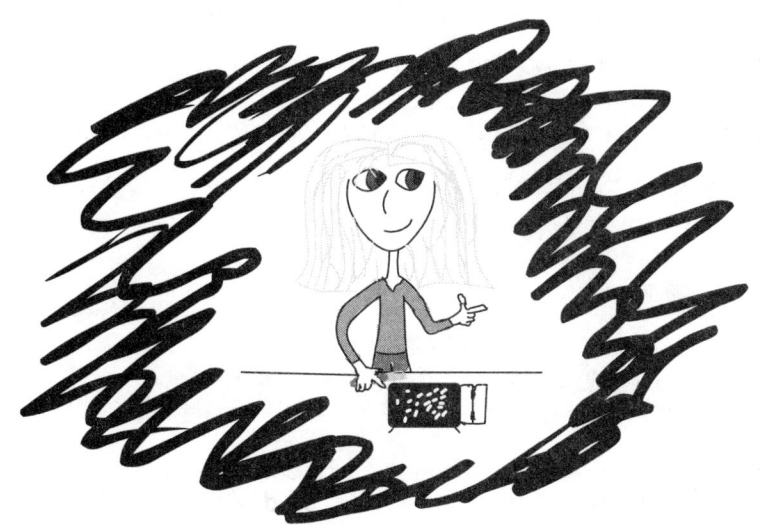

"You may find this hard to believe, but... Watching me doesn't make me go ANY faster!"

Tess Perle is a registered trademark of Salt & Light Enterprises, LLC.

At www.rxtechsuccess.com, you will find great gifts for your favorite technician or yourself!

✂ ✂ ✂ ✂ ✂ ✂ ✂ ✂ ✂ ✂ ✂

Cut here to use order form

Please check box to indicate the products you would like to order:
(Add $6.50 for S&H)

☐	*Rx Success* Compounding Kit and Workbook Upgrade	$249.95
☐	*Rx Success* National Certification Review Manual	$39.95
☐	*Rx Success* Exam Prep Phlash™ Cards	$19.95
☐	*Rx Success* Drug Memorization Phlash™ Cards	$25.95

Allow 2-3 weeks for delivery

Name: _____

Address: _____

Email: _____

Mail Order Form and Check or Money Order to:
Salt & Light Enterprises, LLC
1004 Mockingbird Street
Brighton, Colorado 80601
(866) 898-9374
Makes checks payable to "Salt & Light Enterprises, LLC"